Keto Desserts Cookbook

For Beginners

50 Best Low-Carb And Sugar-Free

Keto Recipes

EMILY EVANS

Keto Desserts Cookbook For Beginners

Table of Contents

Introduction

The ketogenic diet, or keto diet, is a high-fat diet that promotes a healthy lifestyle without any carbs and sugar. A food with super-low or no amount of carbs gets the body into ketosis, which is the primary goal of the ketogenic diet. Ketosis is a metabolic process in which the body switch to fats to get energy when carbs reserves are finished. Following are some proven benefits of the ketogenic diet:

- Weight loss

- Clear skin

- Reduced inflammation

- Mental clarity and focused

- More energy

- Reduced cravings
- Reduce the risk of chronic and metabolic diseases

Let's go into some more details of the ketogenic diet.

As a result, fat is broken down into simpler molecules called

ketones which are transported to body cells to use as fuel. A great benefit of getting your body into ketosis is that when carbs are broken down into sugar, insulin hormone triggers craving and you feel unnecessarily hungry, while when carbs are limited, and fats are increased, these cravings are stopped and hence, your appetite gets into your control completely.So, whatever you eat on a ketogenic diet, be it have carbs or sugar, just make sure that the body stays into ketosis process and don't spike its blood sugar level. Sugar is also a form of carbohydrate, and the amount of carbs allowed for a keto-er is about 50 grams or below this threshold per day. This amount includes refined sugar and all the sources of carbs. So does this mean that you have to cut back on desserts? Absolutely not. Being on the Keto diet, you can still satisfy your sweet tooth and enjoy sweet treats. All you need to do is to prepare those desserts that don't bring your body out of ketosis. And, there are two keys to do this. Firstly, you need to choose keto-friendly ingredients that are high in fats to support ketone formation in the body.

And, secondly, use a sweetener that doesn't spike blood glucose level to critical level. Luckily, there are many sweeteners available in the market that add flavor to your desserts, without increasing carbs and sugar in it.

- Stevia: This natural sweetener is nonnutritive, and this means it has no carbs or calories. Stevia is a great option to control and lower your blood sugar levels. It is available in both powdered and syrup form, but it is much sweeter than table sugar, therefore use less stevia quantity to achieve same sweetness – 1 teaspoon stevia for 1 cup sugar.

- Sucralose: This sucralose based artificial sweetener is indigestible and thus, provide no calories and carbs. Feel free to use this sweetener for any dessert except for those that require baking. Substitute it in the 1:1 ratio for most of the dessert recipes.

- Erythritol: It is a type of sugar alcohol that stimulates your taste buds which give you a taste of sugar. It can substitute sugar in a wide variety of dessert recipes, be it baking or cooking.

- Xylitol: This sugar alcohol is commonly found in gum and candies, and like other keto sweeteners, it has no carbs. Give a kick of flavor to your smoothies, shakes, tea, and coffee with this sweetener. Moreover, it also works well with baked desserts. However, do add a little bit liquid when using xylitol as it absorbs moisture and increases dryness.

Exchange xylitol in a 1:1 ratio with regular sugar. Monk Fruit Sweetener: As the name suggests, this sweetener is extracted from the monk fruit and thus, contain natural sugar.

And, since this extract contains no sugar and calorie, it is an excellent option for a ketogenic diet. Use it anywhere in place of regular sugar. You can also use fruits to add sweetness to your desserts such as:

- Strawberries

- Raspberries

- Blackberries

- Blueberries

- Lemon

- Lime

- Watermelon

- Cherries

- Peach

- Kiwi

- Cantaloupe

- Mandarin

Following are some sweeteners that are high in carbs, and you must avoid them.

- Honey

- Coconut sugar

- Maple syrup

- Agave nectar

- Dates

Here are some more tips that will help you satisfy your sweet tooth.

- It is normal to crave for sugar in the initial days of Ketogenic dieting. You will have temptation for sweet once in a while, and when this happens, Keto-friendly sweeteners

can satisfy your sweet cravings without stalling your fat loss and maintaining the ketosis process in your body.

- Differentiate between the types of sweeteners that are available for the Ketogenic diet.

There are three categories – natural sweeteners, sugar alcohols, and artificial sweeteners. Erythritol and stevia work just perfectly for any desserts without disturbing your insulin and blood sugar.

- Enhance your weight loss with Keto sweeteners. As mentioned before, sugar is also a

form of carb and therefore, using them in an appropriate amount not only led to shedding weight, it also optimizes your health.

What is keto?

The ketogenic diet (as you already know, I am sure) is a diet designed to put the body into a state of ketosis. This is done by **heavily** reducing the number of carbs eaten and increasing the intake of fats. When we eat carbs, our body uses them for energy and stores the excess as glycogen. This means that the fat we eat is stored away as fat (yup, the kinda fat we can see and touch). What's more, when we eat carbs (especially sugars!) our blood sugar spikes. When we **remove** these carbs, our body has to turn to fat as an energy source. When our body starts breaking down fats to use as energy, the liver produces ketones which are also used as energy. And there you have it, a short explanation of the ketosis process.

What you really need to know here (because this book is all about food, after all!) is that the ketogenic diet relies on a specific breakdown of macronutrients (carbs, fats and proteins). The most **crucial** macro to keep an eye on is carbs. The general number most people stick to is 30 grams of net carbs per day. Net carbs is simply the total carbs with the fiber subtracted. You also have to be careful about how much protein you eat too, as too much can actually take you out of ketosis. Many people use this formula for their protein intake while on keto: 0.6 grams of protein per pound of body weight. For example, a 170-pound person would eat 90 grams of protein per day. After a small amount of carbs, the rest of their food intake would be made up of healthy fat.

Many people choose to try the ketogenic to lose weight, especially around the middle. Others try it to increase energy levels, reduce the risk of diabetes or even for fertility purposes. But we will get into the great benefits of the keto diet below!

Interestingly, the ketogenic diet was popular about 100 years ago for the treatment of epilepsy. The ketogenic diet is basically a fancy, calculated way of fasting. Fasting has been used for millennia, as thinkers and holy people fasted as a spiritual practice, but also to boost their energy levels and inspire sharp thinking. That's just a little snippet of history to put the ketogenic diet into context! Fast forward to today, and keto is a popular diet for many people for many reasons, helped along by technology. There are many apps such as MyFitnessPal which calculate the macronutrients in everything you eat, providing you with the correct fat, protein, total carbs, net carbs and calories.

Switching to a Ketogenic Diet:

Ketogenic is not simply a diet; it is a whole lifestyle unlike many misinterpret. Being a lifestyle means that you just not need some dietary changes to get to the perks of the ketosis, you also need to turn your whole routine according to those changes, meaning, keto meal along with routine exercise, hydration, and proper sleep. A combination of all these changes will result in the keto oriented health effects. When a person switches to a ketogenic diet, he or she goes through three important phases:

1. Induction Phase:

Entering into the world of ketogenic diet require more of the mental strength than physical. It is important to prepare your mind for it and then act on it. Thus, the first phase is all about preparing yourself for this special diet. An easy way to do that is by removing all the possible high carb food items from your groceries and opting for more clean carbs. Do your research and plan things out for yourself. Be steadier and more gradual to have a more lasting impact. Start limiting the number of carbs and keep track of the fat's intake. Habit and discipline are most important while surviving through this phase. Loss of will means loss of efforts, so start sticking to the routine.

2. Adjustment Phase:

Now that the induction phase has passed, the adjustment phase allows a person to add more variety to the diet using a variety of keto friendly fruits and vegetables. It is safe to add more fats to the diet through cream, cheeses or vegetable oils. In this phase, the body goes through slight changes in terms of energy levels and health. This adjustment in the diet is important to keep up with the pace of those changes.

3. Fitness Phase:

The last phase is the fitness phase. By this time, the routine for the keto diet must be well developed. However, the body still needs a kick start to burn more fat than glucose. A little exercise is recommended at this stage to help achieve the aim. Such exercise may range from light intensity aerobics to high-intensity exercises. Physical exercises together with a planned ketogenic diet are the road to a healthy and active life. The keto diet triggers the production of ketones inside the body.

These ketone masses are then used as an energy source instead of glucose. The 'keto' part of the ketogenic diet plan is extracted from this. The ketones act as energy sources while the amount of sugar in the body is low.

Carbohydrates intake is inversely proportional to the production of the ketones in the body, meaning the lesser the carb intake, the higher the ketones production. Ketones are not directly produced through food breakdown rather, the processing of fat results in the ketonic production. These ketones are essential for vital brain functions. This is the reason that the first ketogenic diet was used only to cure patients of epilepsy and other brain-related diseases. That is why switching to a ketogenic diet quickly results in better mental health.

Carbohydrates may provide energy instantly, but that amount is not lasting that is why a sugary meal can make your energy levels drain within an hour or so, whereas keto diet provides energy through fat processing and consumption, which is long lasting and much higher than provided through the same amount of carbs.

When Ketogenic Diet is Right for You? These conditions include:

People having type 1 diabetes or taking insulin medications. Ketogenic diet in such cases can cause ketoacidosis which is quite harmful and even fatal.

People having Blood Pressure complications should also ask a professional before opting for ketogenic lifestyle.

Breastfeeding mothers.

Signs that you are on a ketogenic diet:

Many individuals ask when actually the sign of ketosis appears? Having to know it tells you that you are in the right direction and following the diet correctly. Since this diet benefits us more internally than externally for normal people, it is hard to witness the changes easily. There are however certain related signs which help us predict the direction correctly, and those are:

Dry Mouth and Constant Thirst:

Right from the induction phase, ketosis can render more dehydration and requires more water intake than usual. This is why, when a person switches to the diet it gives a constant feeling of thirst. Making your body fat dependent is a major shift, which can cause a temporary electrolyte imbalance as the body molds to adopt it. That is why try to drink as much water as to can on a daily basis.

Increased Urination:

Acetoacetate is the compound which is a ketosis byproduct. It ends up in the urine and produces a constant urge of urination. Moreover, more water intake in the diet also adds up to the frequent urination. These two reasons together can cause an increased rate of urination.

Which is a healthy sign as it allows the toxins to release out of the body more frequently?

Ketogenic breath:

It will be interesting to know for many that when we switch to a ketogenic diet, it also affects our breath and render is smell more fruiter like a nail polish remover. It is mainly because acetone is released out of the body through the mouth. It happens of quite a few days after starting the ketogenic diet whereas it disappears with time. The same smell can be sensed through the body sweat.

High Energy Level:

The most visible sign of a keto diet is elevated levels of energy. The concentration level increases and a person can feel a spark in the body. Such positive energy can last throughout the day both physically and mentally.

Lower Need to Eat:

This happens because the body has shifted from glucose to fats as energy sources. Keto followers are satisfied with eating once or twice a day, and this leads to unconscious intermittent fasting. This aids a lot in losing weight and is very tie saving apart from its financial feasibility.

What are the Perks of a Keto Diet?

The ketogenic diet has numerous advantages due to the selective approach it has. Every meal that we eat is an energy booster that is equally healthy. This is the secret behind the popularity of the keto plan. It has outpaced all other dietary plans in the race due to its rich and healthy content. Let's find out more of its pros before switching to the plan.

Fat Burn

The main objective of a keto diet is to consume fats as a source of energy instead of carbohydrates. Therefore, when a person is on a keto diet, more fats present in the body are burnt which consequently reduced weight and prevents obesity.

Lower Cholesterol:

Consumption of fats in the energy-producing process means reduced cholesterol levels in the blood. This is particularly important for patients suffering from cardiovascular diseases and higher cholesterol levels.

Lower Blood Sugar:

Diabetes or high blood sugar level is caused due to zero or minimum production of insulin hormone in the body. People suffering from such disorder cannot regulate their blood sugar levels naturally, therefore, they need a diet low on sugars, and ketogenic is one best option for such individuals.

Increased Energy:

A single fats molecule can produce three times more energy than a carbohydrate when broken down. This is the reason that the use of the ketogenic diet gives us an instant and long-lasting boost of energy after a meal.

VITALITY:

Though scientists are still trying to bring out direct evidence of the effects of ketogenic diet on the increased vitality of a person, they are however sure to say that keto food improves health in the longer run, aides an active metabolism and detoxifies the body regularly, which all can lead to increased vitality.

Mental focus:

While it is true that the ketogenic diet originally came to use for the treatment of mental illnesses like epilepsy and Alzheimer etc. it is also true that lesser consumption of carbohydrates and more availability of ketones in the body, detoxify the blood and nourished neural cells.

Reduce obesity:

There is a huge misconception that intake of more fats can cause obesity. It is true when you take fats along with excessive carbohydrates. Along with fats like that in keto diet does not cause obesity instead it reduces it by consuming all the deposited fats in the body.

METABOLISM:

Increased energy production through ketosis leads to better metabolism. Due to the presence of fat molecules in the food, the bodywork rigorously during and after the digestion to generate energy.

Additional Benefits:

- It is great for the skin and helps it fight against the acne problems.
- Reduces the sensation of heart burning.

- It aids the body to fight against brain cancer.
- Reduces the rate of migraine attacks.
- Lowers the level of sugar in the blood and prevents its addiction.
- Treats ALZHEIMER'S disease.

What to Eat on a Ketogenic Diet?

To make things simple and easier, let's break it down a little and try to understand the Keto vegetarian diet plan as a chart explaining what to have and what not to have. Down below is a brief list of all the items which can be used on a Ketogenic vegetarian diet.

• All Meats:

All types of meat are free from carbohydrates, so it is always safe to use meat in the ketogenic diet. However, processed meat which may contain high traces of carbohydrates should be avoided.

• Selective Vegetables:

Keep this in mind that not all vegetables are low on carbs. There are some who are full of starch, and they need to be avoided. A simple technique to access the suitability of the vegetables for a keto diet is to check if they are 'grown above the ground' or 'below it.' All vegetables which are grown underground are a no go for Keto whereas vegetables which are grown above are best for keto and these mainly include cauliflower, broccoli, zucchini, etc. Among the vegetables, all the leafy green vegetables can be added to this diet which includes spinach, kale, parsley, cilantro, etc.

• Dry Nuts and Seeds etc.:

Nuts and seeds like sunflower seeds, pistachios, pumpkin seeds, almonds, etc. can all be used on a ketogenic diet.

• Selective Dairy:

Not every dairy product is allowed on a keto diet. For example, milk is a no-go for keto whereas hard cheeses, high fat cream, butter, eggs, etc. can all be used.

• Keto friendly Fruits:

Not all berries are Keto friendly, only choose blackberries or raspberries, and other low carb berries. Similarly, not all fruits can be taken on a keto diet, avocado, coconut, etc. are keto friendly whereas orange, apples, and pineapple, etc. are high in carbohydrates.

• All Fats:

Ghee, butter, plant oils, animal fats all forms of fats can be used on a ketogenic diet.

• Keto substitute:

As sugar is strictly forbidden for a ketogenic diet, may it be brown or white there is a certain substitute which can be used like:

1. Stevia

2. Erythritol

3. Swerve

4. monk fruit,

5. Natvia

6. other low-carb sweeteners

What to Avoid on Keto Diet?Avoiding carbohydrate is the main aim of a ketogenic diet. Most of the daily items we use contain a high amount of carbohydrates in the form of sugars or starch. In fact, any amount these items drastically increase the carbohydrate value of your meal. So, it is best to avoid their use completely.

1. All Grains including Rice and Wheat:

All types of grains are high in carbohydrates, whether its rice or corn or wheat. And product extracting out them is equally high in carbs, like corn flour, wheat flour or rice flour. So, while you need to avoid these grains for keto, their flours should also be avoided. Coconut and almond flours can be used as a good substitute.

2. All Legumes including lentils and beans:

Legumes are also the underground parts of the plants; thus, they are highly rich in carbohydrates. Make no mistake of using them in your diet. These include all sorts of beans, from Lima to chickpeas, Garbanzo, black, white, red beans, etc. cross all of them off your grocery list if you are about to go keto. All types of lentils are also not allowed on a keto diet.

3. Every natural and synthetic Sugar:

Besides white and brown sugar there are other forms of it which are also not keto friendly, this list includes honey, agave, molasses, maple syrup, etc. Also, avoid chocolates which are high in sugar. Use special sweeteners and sugar-free chocolates only.

4. High Carb Fruits:

Certain fruits need to be avoided while on a keto diet. Apples, bananas, oranges, pineapple, etc. all fall into that category. Do not use them in any form. Avoid using their flesh, juice, and mash to keep your meal carb free.

5. Underground Tubers:

Tubers are basically underground vegetables, and some of them are rich in carbs including potatoes, yams, sweet potatoes, beets, etc.

6. Animal Milk:

As stated above, not all dairy product can be freely used on a ketogenic diet. Animal milk should be strictly avoided.

What are the benefits

Weight loss

The number one reason why modern people choose to try the ketogenic diet is weight loss. When you eat a high-fat diet, you become satiated and full much sooner than you would with a high-carb or low-fat diet. This helps you to eat smaller portions and therefore fewer calories over time. What's more, by cutting out sugary, starchy foods and replacing them with wholesome, veggie-based foods, you cut out **lots** of calories. The very nature of the ketogenic diet means that the body turns into a fat burning machine, helping to tap into stored fat, leaving you feeling slenderer and leaner! The ketogenic diet also really helps to regulate and boost your insulin sensitivity, which helps with weight loss and vice versa (losing excess weight helps with insulin issues such as insulin resistance!).

Abundant energy and sharper mind

So many keto dieters find that one of the very best side effects is increased energy levels and a sharp mind. The ketones that your body produces while burning fat for energy are actually an awesome source of energy for your brain. This means that your brain works harder, faster and sharper! Get more work done, win any argument and generally feel sharp as a tack.

Disease prevention

The ketogenic diet could help your body to stave off certain diseases such as diabetes, metabolic disease, cancer and even Alzheimer's disease. The ketogenic diet helps to regulate blood sugar levels and weight, both of which are really important factors for health and longevity. By eating lots of healthy fats and nutritious veggies, your heart is also supported! However, it's important to choose healthy fats (avocado, nuts, seeds, cold pressed oils and fish) as opposed to filling yourself with butter, cream and animal fats. By cutting out processed sugars and starchy carbs and replacing them with nutrient-dense plant-based foods and grass-fed meats, your body has a much better chance at functioning at optimal level for decades, with a far lower risk of developing diseases.

Great for the skin

If you approach your keto diet with a healthy mindset and focus on nutrition as well as macros, you'll likely find that your skin becomes clear and glowy. High-fat foods (healthy fats, that is) such as avocados, nuts, seeds, olive oil, flaxseed oil and oily fish are all incredible for the skin. They nourish and hydrate the skin from the inside, leaving you with a healthy, youthful and luminous complexion.

Takes care of blood sugar levels

When you eat sugar and carbs, your blood sugar goes a little wonky. In fact, it spikes and increases. When this happens over and over again, you risk all kinds of complications such as type 2 diabetes and obesity. Out-of-whack blood sugar levels can make you feel sleepy, dizzy and generally not so great. The ketogenic diet can really help to stabilize your blood sugar, helping you to feel energetic and on top of the world. In fact, this is one of the main medical reasons why the ketogenic is recommended!

Keto Side Effects

At this point you might be wondering what kind of toll such a significant change to your diet is going to take on how you feel, especially if you are used to consuming higher amounts of carbohydrates. Your body may have built up a stock of carbohydrate-active enzymes, and therefore might not be well-equipped to break down and store large volumes of fat, or to deal with a sudden shortage of glucose. As a result, your body has to produce an entirely new supply of enzymes. After an adjustment period, your body will naturally begin to use your reserves of glucose, stored in the liver and muscles, for energy. This can lead to lethargy and sluggishness.Many people cite dizziness, headaches and irritability as early side effects of the keto diet, particularly during the first seven days. This is due to the depletion of electrolytes from your system, which is, of course, another reason to drink plenty of fluids and replenish your sodium levels. As a matter of fact, since sodium helps retain water in the body, many dieticians recommend upping your salt intake significantly.

The keto flu: We've already mentioned the keto flu, but as it is one of the most common side effects of the keto diet, let's examine it in a little more detail. Despite the name, the keto flu (also known as the 'low-carb flu') is not actually a kind of influenza. It is so-called because many newcomers to the keto diet experience a number of flu-like symptoms in the early stages of their keto transformation.

There are two main reasons why the keto flu occurs:

1. More frequent trips to the bathroom: Increased urination leads to a considerable loss of electrolytes and water. You can preemptively combat this problem by drinking a bouillon cube dissolved in water.

2. Withdrawal: Remember, your body is going through a major transition! It now has to adjust to a significant drop in carb intake and create new enzymes in order to process increased amounts of fat. This is hard work for your body, and you may feel lethargic as

a result. To ease this, you should try decreasing your carb intake gradually, rather than quitting cold turkey.

Increasing your water consumption and replacing lost electrolytes will effectively combat or even eradicate the keto flu. At the beginning of your transition you should try to eat less than 15 grams of carbohydrates a day, then decrease this number little by little over time.

Nothing worth doing is easy, but thankfully the drawbacks of the keto diet are few and, for the most part, easily alleviated. The same cannot be said for many other fad diets out there!

Here are some other notable side effects of the ketogenic diet, and suggestions as to how you can deal with them.

- Fatigue and irritability – High ketone levels can positively impact your physical wellbeing in a number of ways, but they are also linked to increased tiredness and quicker exertion during exercise. Make sure you are getting enough sleep during the early days of your transition and avoid particularly strenuous exercise if necessary.

- 'Brain fog' – Your altered metabolism and hormonal state may cause decreased mental clarity or 'brain fog.' This is a common side effect of total carbohydrate withdrawal, which is why you should avoid going cold turkey and instead decrease your carbohydrate intake gradually and steadily.

- Change in lipids – An important tenet of the ketogenic diet is not only to up your fat intake but also to watch what kinds of fats you are consuming. Saturated fats are known to increase cholesterol levels, so make sure they do not outbalance the non- saturated fats in your diet.

- Micronutrient deficiencies – Low-carb foods are often lacking in important nutrients like magnesium, potassium and iron. Taking supplements is an excellent way of compensating for this.

- Ketoacidosis – If your diet is poorly-planned, you may be at risk of developing ketoacidosis, which is characterized by extremely high ketone levels. This is especially harmful to sufferers of diabetes, so make sure you organize your diet so as

to keep your ketone levels within a healthy range. Additionally, it is important to know how to recognize the signs. These include a shortness of breath, pain in the abdomen, confusion, nausea, vomiting, and weakness. If you experience any combination of these symptoms while on the ketogenic diet, seek medical attention immediately.

- Muscle loss – Decreased carbohydrate consumption means your body may draw on protein in your muscles for energy, leading to a decrease in muscle mass. In particular this side effect is associated with those who engage in rigorous workouts, so consider scaling back your exercise routine if muscle loss is a major concern for you.

Chapter 1:

List of ingredients used for keto desserts.

The keto-friendly "YES" foods: these are the low-carb foods which are permitted on the ketogenic diet. Some of them can be eaten liberally, such as leafy greens. Others can be eaten with a little more moderation, such as nuts and berries. Your calorie counter/macro calculator will let you know exactly how many net carbs are in each food, so you will soon learn the right quantities and it will become second nature!

Oils:

- Olive oil Avocado oil Flaxseed oil MCT oil Coconut oil
- Walnut oil Nuts and seeds:
- Almonds
- Walnuts
- Pecans

- Brazil nuts Hazelnuts Macadamia nuts Cashews Pumpkin seeds
- Sunflower seeds
- Chia seeds Sesame seeds
- Nut and seed butters

(plain, no flavors or sugars added) Low carb veggies:

- Lettuce Spinach Kale
- Avocado (technically a fruit...but it's an **incredible** keto food, full of healthy fats and fiber)
- Asparagus
- Artichokes Cabbage Broccoli Cauliflower Bok choy Chard Celery Green beans Mushrooms
- Mustard greens Tomatoes Zucchini Spaghetti squash
- Mung beans Cucumber
- Berries in moderation:

All berries are fine, but raspberries and blackberries have fewer carbs than strawberries and blueberries, so keep that in mind. Just stick to a small portion of berries and you'll be fine!

Eggs and soy proteins:

Free range eggs are a great source of fat and protein without any carbs Tofu and tempeh are great protein sources for vegans and vegetarians Grass-fed meats:

Choose organic, grass-fed meats. As long as there are no seasonings or marinades added, you can enjoy all forms of meat. Ground meat, steaks, roasts, chops, legs... it's all good!

Bacon Beef Pork Venison Lamb

Fish and poultry:

All fish and poultry is 100% permitted as long as it's not pre-seasoned or marinated Choose free range poultry and wild-caught fish

Salmon is a fantastic choice because it's full of healthy fats and oils Salmon

Tuna

All white fish

Chicken Turkey

Full fat dairy:

Full-fat cream

Full-fat plain, unsweetened yogurt (NO low fat or fat free varieties allowed!) Full-fat sour cream

Full-fat ricotta

Full-fat mascarpone Cheese:

Cheddar Brie Camembert Blue cheese

Parmesan cheese

Feta cheese Goat cheese Colby cheese

Keto sweetener: Stevia

Erythritol Xylitol

Herbs and spices:

All fresh and dried herbs are completely permitted

Use dried spices to flavor your food, just beware of mixed seasonings and rubs as they can often contain sugar

Keto flours:

Coconut flour

Almond flour/ground almonds Ground flaxseed

Ground hazelnuts Coffee and tea:

Add cream to your coffee for a fat booster!

NO sugar in that cup of hot tea! Use a sweetener such as Stevia instead

NO milk in your tea and coffee, always use cream as milk contains sugar Alcohol:

All spirits are okay on keto, in moderation. Note: this does **not** include liqueurs or sugary drinks such as Kahlua or Baileys Irish Cream. Plain, pure spirits such as vodka, gin, whiskey, rum and tequila are all zero-carb as long as you mix them with water, plain soda or zero-carb soda.

Champagne, dry white wine and red wine are all fine in moderation. For example, one glass of champagne (around 5oz) has a maximum of 2 grams of net carbs.

Mixers: plain, unflavored soda with fresh citrus is best Sauces and condiments:

Full-fat mayonnaise and fresh guacamole are permitted the keto diet as long as they do not contain sugar. Salad dressing made from oil and vinegar is fine, but watch out for store-bought salad dressings which are often packed with sugar.

The keto-banned "NO WAY" foods:

Pasta, noodles, bread and rice:

All pasta, noodles, bread and rice are off limits. Basically, anything made from flour or grains is out of bounds.

Beans, lentils, chickpeas: Unfortunately, beans, lentils and chickpeas are all prohibited on the keto diet because of their high carb content. These foods are in the legume food group and are all banned on keto. This also includes peas and peanuts.

Baked goods:

Traditional baked goods such as cakes, cookies, bars, breads, scones and cupcakes are all out of the question on keto. If they contain flour and sugar, get rid of them.

Sugary treats:

Candy, chocolate (except 72% cocoa dark chocolate), ice cream and all things in the candy aisle are not allowed on keto. If you're craving a sweet treat, pick a recipe from this book!

Juice, soda, premixed alcoholic drinks:

Fruit juices, sodas and premixed alcoholic drinks ("alcopops") are filled with sugar and are not ketogenic-approved. Stick to water, plain soda water, tea and coffee.

Grains:

Grains such as rice, quinoa, oats and barley are all ruled out on keto because they are high-carb foods. You can use cauliflower and broccoli as rice substitutes.

Milk:

Milk contains sugar and is therefore not permitted on keto. Stick to full-fat cream or unsweetened nut milks such as almond milk.

Most fruits:

The only fruits you can eat on keto are avocados and berries (in moderation). Avoid all other fruits, especially bananas. Fruits are high-carb, high-sugar foods. While fruits are not unhealthy, they're simply too carb-rich and therefore negate the ketogenic process.

Starchy veggies:

Starchy veggies such as potato, sweet potato, corn, yams, peas, carrots and beets are not keto- friendly as they are high in carbs. Stick to leafy greens and low-carb veggies as listed above.

Sauces and condiments:

Stay away from store-bought sauces, condiments and marinades as they are often packed with sugars. Make your own dressings, sauces and marinades at home so you know exactly what's in them.

Tips for choosing the right keto foods

- Check the labels on any packaged foods. Does it contain sugar? Put it back! Does it have a high net carb count? Put it back!

- Try to choose foods which are close to the source and haven't been processed or packaged. Think meat, eggs, nuts/seeds, veggies, full-fat diary, oils etc.

- Install a calorie-counter app on your phone so you can always check the macros of any food if you're unsure

- Does it contain flour, sugar or starchy veggies? No go!

- Keep an eye on your portion sizes. If one portion is perfectly balanced with the right amount of carbs, an extra portion may tip you over the edge. If you're still hungry after dinner? Fill up on a fresh salad with an olive oil dressing

Can you really eat dessert on keto?

Keto isn't about cutting out certain meals or recipes...it's about sticking to the correct macros. This means that as long as your dessert is within the parameters of your macros, it's completely permitted! Luckily for us, ingredients such as butter, cream, sour cream, mascarpone, cream cheese and eggs are all wonderfully keto-friendly foods...and perfect dessert ingredients too.

When it comes to sugar, there are many non-sugar sweeteners out there which are 100% keto approved. Stevia, erythritol and xylitol are the most popular sweeteners as they don't spike the blood sugar at all.

I think that Stevia is the best sweetener as you only need a very small amount and it contains barely any carbs or calories.

Note: these recipes were all formulated using STEVIA which is extremely sweet and only requires 1 tsp per 1 cup of regular sugar. Other sweeteners are less sweet and require a far larger measure. My advice is to use Stevia for these recipes to get the best result.

Concerned about the issue of flour? No worries! We use ground almonds and sometimes ground hazelnuts. Ground almonds provide awesome fat and protein, with more fiber than regular flour. Ground almonds do give a denser result, but to me, that's a great thing! A dense, fudgy cake is nothing to be mad about.

Keto dessert ingredient staples (staples in these recipes, at least!)

- Heavy cream
- Real butter (grass-fed butter, no margarine or butter substitutes please!)
- Coconut oil, canola oil, olive oil, flaxseed oil
- Cocoa powder (unsweetened, always)
- Pure vanilla extract (no essence or imitations)
- Fresh mint
- Flavor essences (such as almond or caramel)
- Cream cheese (plain, full fat)
- Espresso powder
- Mascarpone cheese (plain, full fat)
- Keto sweeteners such as Stevia

- Almonds, hazelnuts and walnuts (ground and whole)

- Salt (for bringing out chocolate flavor)

- Eggs (always free range)

- Berries (frozen, fresh and freeze-dried)

- Lemon zest and juice

- 72% cocoa dark chocolate (a small amount, and it must be at least 72% cocoa!)

How to know if you have achieved ketosis

There are various ways with which you can find out whether you are in ketosis or not. Some of them are as following-

Keto Strip test

It is a common way to find out whether you are in ketosis or not. Keto strips tell you the level of ketones your body is getting rid of.

Blood glucose test

This test lets you know your glucose levels. Increased urination When in Ketosis you will go to the loo more than before because Keto is a natural diuretic. It will get normal in a few days.

Dry mouth

When you enter Ketosis, you will find that your body will release more fluids and it will require more electrolytes, because of this you will experience dry mouth. It will happen only for few days, than you will be perfectly normal.

Bad breath

Acetone is a ketone that is partially excreted through your breath. You might find bad breath for few days, than it will get perfectly fine.

Reduced hunger. You will not find yourself hungry all the time like in other diets. When you are in ketosis, your hunger goes down and you don't have to eat all the time.

Increased energy
You will find that you energy levels will increase when you enter ketosis.

Exercise on a ketogenic diet

On Ketogenic diet people can lose weight without exercising. Everyone would love to lose fat without exercising and changing their lifestyle. All you have to do is change your eating habits and rest will be taken care of.

Working out on a keto diet
You will not experience a loss of physical performance when you are on ketogenic diet. You can easily exercise if you want to and you should workout for greater benefits.

Worries
Most people believe that carbohydrates provide with energy required for workouts, this is true but when you are following Ketogenic diet you cannot eat more than 50 grams of carbohydrates, how can your body survive the workouts when you are not eating enough carbohydrates?

Having these doubts are justified but the best news is that your body does not require carbohydrates at all when in the state of ketosis, your body will use ketones as a source of energy which is your fat in your body. How awesome will that be, getting energy from fats to burn off fat. When you are in Ketosis, your body will burn sugar first which is in your body, it will use all the sugar and then switch to fats for its energy source.

Ketosis

When you are in ketosis your energy levels will increase, and your body will not require carbohydrates at all. But if you have just started your ketogenic diet, than you might feel little tired, so it is best to take few carbohydrates before your workouts or avoid exercise during first week of ketogenic diet so that your body completely adapts to ketogenic diet.

Eating a lot.

People who are active generally have higher metabolism than those who are less active. This also means that people who have higher metabolism will eat more food than those who have lower metabolism.

Sometimes people eat too much on this diet thinking that you can eat as much as you want in this diet and then they don't see any weight change, they start blaming the diet. Yes, it is important to eat and refuel your body but at the same time you should make sure that you are eating the right amount based on your macros. This is where majority of people go wrong. Either they eat too much and don't see any results or they eat too less and become demotivated and annoyed with the diet. Finding the right size is important in this diet.

Many times people will eat too much after their workouts, they feel like they need to stuff their face after the workout but only if they show little discipline they can achieve miracles.

You will count your macros based on your activity levels. If you live a very active lifestyle then you are allowed to eat more but if you are not very active than you should try to eat less and this is same in all types of diets.

Weight Loss

Ketogenic diet main purpose is to make you slim, if you add exercise with your diet than you will be able to lose enormous amount of weight. You should combine the two i.e. diet and exercise for best results.

Your number on the weighing machine will drop faster than compared to if you were not exercising.

Again I would like to tell you that exercise is not necessary in Ketogenic lifestyle but it will increase the speed of fat loss for sure.

Performance will not suffer
Many people these days have this misconception about Ketogenic diet that if you are on Ketogenic diet than your performance in gym will go down. This is not true at all.

Yes in beginning, your performance might go down a little bit but in the long run your performance will be much better than what it used to be on normal diet.

Tests have been done on athletes before and after being on Keto diet and the results are that athletes performed better while being on keto diet.

If you want to workout on keto diet than go for it, don't let false doubts and myths get to you.

Just follow the macros, in Ketogenic diet, food is more important than workout, so make sure you hit your macros.

Macros

Macros is the short form of macronutrients (fats, proteins and carbohydrates). These macros are the basis of calories that you consume.

Calculating your macronutrients and total calories are very important on Ketogenic diet. First calculating macros will look really tough, but it is actually really easy once you understand it.

Everyone is different so macros are different for everyone. Total calories are different for everyone. Those who live really active lifestyle will consume more calories than those who don't work out at all.

When calculating macros, the first step is to calculate your TDEE (Total Daily Energy Expenditure). It is basically total number of calories that you burn in a day. If you eat less than your total daily energy expenditure than you will lose weight, but if you eat more than your total daily energy expenditure than you will gain weight.

BASIC FORMULA

In this formula first we will calculate your resting energy expenditure, that is energy required to run your body when you don't move at all.

For males

10 x weight (kg) + 6.24 x height (cm) – 5 x (age) + 6 = Resting energy expenditure. For females

10 x weight (kg) + 6.24 x height (cm) – 5 x (age) – 159 = Resting energy expenditure.

Since most people do move and not just lie in their bed, next we have to find expenditure of their movements.

Sedentary

Walking, talking, eating etc. Normal day to day mundane activities. (REE x 1.1)

Light activity

Activities which burn around 200-400 calories for women and 250-500 calories for men comes under light activity. (REE x 1.38)

Moderate activity

Activities which burns 400-650 calories for women and 500-800 calories for men comes under moderate activity. (REE x 1.6).

Very active

Activities which burn more than 651 calories for women and more than 801 calories for men comes under very active.(REE x 1.8).

A typical TDEE equation is like this

Let's say you are 30 years old, 184 cm, 90 kgs, very active man These will be your results

(10 x weight (kg) + 6.24 x height (cm) − 5 x age (y) + 6 = REE) x 1.8

= TDEE 10 x 90 + 6.24 x 184 − 5 x 30 + 6 = REE

900 + 1148.16 − 150 + 6 = REE

1904.16 = REE

1904.16 x 1.8 = 3427.488

TDEE = 3427.488

If your Total daily energy expenditure is 3427.488. If you will eat more than this, you will gain weight.

If you eat exactly 3427 calories than you will neither lose weight nor will you gain weight. If you will eat less than 3427 calories then you will lose weight for sure.

Losing weight.

If you want to lose weight than I will recommend don't drop your calories more than 20 % of your total daily energy expenditure. This way you will have enough energy to carry out your mundane tasks and live life with ease. You will stick to your diet but if you drop your calories too much than you will become demotivated and irritated by this diet and you will find yourself binge eating.

Gaining weight

Same goes with gaining weight, increase your calories by 20 %. This way you will gain lean muscles and will stay in control of your life.

MACROS

First step was getting your TDEE. Now we will calculate macronutrients that make up your diet. 1gram of protein = 4 calories.

1 gram of fat = 9 calories.

1 gram of carbohydrates = 4 calories.

So suppose you want to lose weight and your TDEE is 2000 calories per day. You will consume around 1600 calories (2000 – 20 % of 2000).

FATS

Now 70 % of 1600 will be from fats. 70 % of 1600 =1120.

1120 / 9 = 125 grams (1 gram of fats = 9 calories) 1120 Calories of fats means 124 grams of fats.

PROTEINS

25 % will be from proteins.

So 25 % of 1600 = 400 calories.

400/4 = 100 grams of proteins will be consumed. CARBOHYDRATES

5% OF 1600 calories will be from carbohydrates which will be around 80 grams of carbohydrates.

But try to lower your carbohydrate intake overtime, it should get below 50 grams per day.

Tools you need to start do homemade desserts

Since you can't buy as many baked goods or treats, you'll be baking a lot more to get your fix. What supplies should you be sure to have? Here's our recommendations:

Measuring cups

Most people have these, but if you don't, order some now. You'll want a full set (1 cup, ½ cup, ⅓ cup, ¼ cup) that's easy to clean and durable. Something cheap is probably fine, you don't really need to get anything fancy.

Measuring spoons

Like measuring cups, whatever is cheap and works for you is acceptable. Metal will probably last longer than plastic, but it's up to you.

Liquid measuring jug

This is a bit different than a regular measuring cup, since it's meant for measuring liquid. A 4-cup jug works for most people, with clear lines. Make sure it's microwave-safe, too.

Kitchen scale

Why bother with a kitchen scale when you have measuring cups and spoons? Baking is a science and even just a tablespoon too much or less can make a difference. To make sure you're adding just enough, use a scale. Many recipes will give you the grams, liters, and so on of an ingredient, along with the cups or tablespoons. When choosing a scale, get one that fits in your kitchen and is easy to use. You should also consider how much weight you want it to be able to hold, since some small ones are limited.

Cookie sheets

There are a lot of cookie sheets out there and the only recommendation we have is to get one that has a rim. This distributes the heat a bit better than a totally-flat sheet and lets you prepare recipes like keto-friendly toffee, other candies, and no-bake desserts you freeze and slice. You should also make sure it's made from aluminum, which is the best material for a cookie sheet.

Round cake pans

For layer cakes and breads, you need round cake pans. There are a variety of sizes, like 6-inch or 9- inch, so consider getting a set. Mini cake pans are also a great idea, since they let you make individual single-serve cakes instead of one big one.

Loaf pan

If you plan on making breads at all, a loaf pan is a good buy. These are rectangular and often deeper than a cake pan. There are glass, ceramic, nonstick, and metal pans. Which one is best depends on your personal taste, though metal ones last longer and breads tend to bake better in aluminum- coated steel.

Silicon molds

Why get molds instead of a regular muffin tin? Silicon molds are very easy to use and sticking isn't a problem, so you don't have to waste parchment paper. You can make a wide variety of foods both sweet and savory in the molds, too. Some people say that silicon infuses baked goods with a weird flavor, while others don't notice anything at all, so you'll have to try it to see for yourself. Silicon molds are safe to use in the oven, dishwasher, and freezer. Having the right baking supplies makes baking much easier and can expand the range of recipes you're able to make.

Microplane

A microplane grater is ideal for zesting ingredients like lemon, lime, orange, ginger, nutmeg, and even nuts and chocolate. These fresh zests add tremendous flavor to both sweet and savory foods, so a microplane is a multipurpose tool. Don't confuse a microplane for a zester; they are different. A zester is thinner with fewer holes, and designed primarily for citrus.

KitchenAid mixer

You really can't beat a KitchenAid mixer for an all-around workhorse. They last forever and are up for anything, especially when you have a selection of attachable whisks. While not the cheapest kitchen tool, they're a great investment and you can frequently find sales.

If you don't have a KitchenAid mixer and you plan on baking, get one as soon as possible. We're saying that as people who bake; KitchenAid did not pay us to say that.

Ice cream maker

This may seem like a specialized tool, and while it is, you'll be very glad to have your own ice cream maker if you're serious about the keto diet and love ice cream. While you can't use cow's milk on the keto diet, you can make ice cream with ingredients like heavy cream, coconut milk, and keto-friendly sweeteners. If you don't want to get another bulky piece of equipment, KitchenAid does have an ice-cream attachment that can makes up to 2 quarts of ice cream. You can also find very affordable ice cream makers in smaller sizes from brands like Hamilton Beach.

Chapter 2:

Time saving tips and the essentials in general

So, you reached your ideal weight. What now? Here are a few tricks you might not know. I maintain my ideal weight for years by simply rotating low-carb days with higher carb days. It works for most people, including me, so you can try this method too. A typical week may consist of three low-carb days, two moderate-carb days and two high-carb days. You can add more protein i.e. more calories to your meals while keeping your carbs low. Further, you can eat a little more carbs only before and after a workout. Once you lose weight, you should go slowly and raise your daily carb intake by 10 - 20 grams during the next two weeks. Your body needs time to adapt to new BMI. In this phase, opt for nutrient-dense food such as potatoes and bananas and avoid processed food. In fact, real food will satiate your taste buds and help you feel fuller; consequently, you will eat fewer calories. Further, you can try LCHF, Paleo, or low-carb Mediterranean diet. You can combine your diet with intermittent fasting and muscle-gaining programs, too. The secret is to find that perfect diet and workout plan that work for your lifestyle, age, body type, and activity level. Yes, sure you can eat dessert and still be healthy and fit. There are so many pitfalls, but you can learn to avoid them along the way. Trust me, I did it.

Quick and easy dessert ideas. A refreshing yogurt parfait with nuts and some shaved keto chocolate is ideal for dessert or snack. It is healthy and loaded with heart-healthy ingredients. In general, Greek yogurt will work wonders as a protein-packed, low-calorie base for your favorite desserts such as fruit salads, frozen yogurt, ice pops, or yogurt bark. If you like creamy cakes, switch them out for a piece of cheesecake. A peanut or sesame butter in combination with fruits are sweet enough to stop sugar cravings; just make sure to avoid super-sweet fruits such as figs, bananas, canned and dried fruits. A smoothie with full-fat milk, peanut butter and some berries makes a great breakfast or dessert; not only it can satisfy your sweet teeth, but it also provides a good serving of protein and fiber; you can freeze leftovers and indulge in great popsicle treats later. An avocado and cacao mousse makes a great go-to snack for you and your kids. Other guilt-free options include flavored Greek yogurt, frozen yogurt, sorbet, hot chocolate, and dark chocolate. A homemade chocolate bar is actually my favorite go-to dessert because I can bring it with me wherever I go – to work, to the gym, on travel, etc. The intensity of unsweetened chocolate makes it easier for me to be satisfied with a small portion.

Balance your diet. Opt for a healthy main course (for instance, choose grilled meat instead of fried fish, and a nutrient-dense side dish instead of chips). Later, you can treat yourself with dessert.

Drink lots of water. Some experts claim that dehydration can cause sugar cravings. Next time you crave that chocolate, drink a glass of water and wait a minute or two. After that, you will eat a small, healthy dessert instead of big piece of the pie.

Eat mindfully. When you feel the urge to dig a spoon into that chocolate cake with buttercream frosting, step back and find a healthier way to satisfy a sweet tooth. Do not let those little treats ruin your hard-earned results with the ketogenic diet. Try eating fresh fruits such as berries; they are nature's candy and they can fill your cravings in most cases.

Listen to your body. You should recognize your main diet pitfalls such as liquid calories, extreme calorie reduction, skipping meals, stressing out about your diet, turning to emotional eating.

Reduce, don't eliminate desserts. Think about cutting your favorite dessert in half. Avoid sneaky liquid calories in cocktails and sodas and you are more likely to take off these pounds. Share your dessert with your dining companion. I can't explain but eating dessert with my partner just tastes better.

Eat fiber-rich food. Fiber is one of the key nutrients that keeps you full longer. If you're trying to shed some pounds, fiber is a must!

Indulge in a keto dessert for breakfast. According to recent studies, eating a "dessert breakfast" may help you speed up weight loss. First and foremost, it will reduce your sugar cravings. Then, your metabolism is most active in the morning. And last but not least, you will regulate ghrelin hormone ("hunger hormone") levels.

Go workout. Exercise is one of the most important components of a healthy lifestyle, according to science. You should be exercising at least 3 times per week. To live an active lifestyle, you do not have to go to the gym; simply try to incorporate exercise into your daily routine. Some fun things you can do include going for a walk, taking the stairs, playing with kids and pets, gardening, cycling, and so forth. Eat a good post-workout dessert to help with recovery; opt for high-protein foods such as whey protein, eggs, protein bars, nuts, peanut butter, chia seeds, and avocado.

Finally, yet importantly, in addition to a well-balanced diet, there are a few additional habits that may contribute to your health. They include moving, cooking at home, taking vacation, taking time for yourself, and good night's sleep. If you are looking for healthy ways to indulge your sweet tooth, this recipe collection may be your go-to source for the healthiest desserts ever.

Baking tips

Even if you were an experienced baker before you went on the keto diet, there are some challenges that might come up. Keto baking is a bit different than regular baking because of the different flours and sweeteners, so there will always be a learning curve. Here are five of the most important tips to remember:

Tip #1: Follow recipes other people have perfected

If you want to make chocolate chip cookies, you could just substitute flours and sweeteners in a recipe you already have, but it may not turn out quite right. When in doubt, look up a keto cookie recipe already tested by another baker. This way, you don't waste ingredients and end up disappointed with the final result. If you really like experimenting and perfecting your own recipes, by all means, play around with keto-friendly flours and sweeteners. If you just want to get those cookies as quickly as possible, follow a recipe that's already keto.

Tip #2: Choose your flours based on what fits the recipe best

You could, in theory, use any type of grain-free flour with any recipe, as long as you follow the correct ratios.

However, certain flours just work better with certain recipes. As an example, you may not want to use coconut flour for a baked good that's meant to be light and fluffy, since coconut flour bakes more densely because of its high fiber content. That's why it's often combined with another type of flour. If you love baking a wide variety of treats and bread, stock your pantry with multiple grain-free flours.

Tip #3: Embrace keto-friendly flavorings

Nut flours and keto-friendly sweeteners can add different tastes to baked goods. You may not always love the result. To mask potentially unpleasant flavors and aftertastes, embrace spices and keto-friendly extracts like vanilla.

You can pretty easily increase the amount of these ingredients and even just a little extra can go a long way. Add more cinnamon to your cookies, brown your grass-fed butter, or add some fresh citrus zest. These flavors will come forward more and you won't taste the nut flours or sweeteners as much.

Baking on the keto diet can be a learning process, so follow tips like looking up tested recipes before creating your own, and always greasing your pans well to master keto baking more quickly.

Tip #4: Prep the ingredients according to the recipe

This is really just a good baking tip - everyone should follow it, whether they're on the keto diet or not. The temperature and texture of ingredients really matter in baking. As we've said before, it's a pretty exact science.

If a recipe says that the eggs should be room temperature, make sure they are room temperature. The same goes for butter and whether or not a flour should be sifted. These may seem like small details, but they make a big difference in baking.

Tip #5: Grease your pans well

Keto baking doesn't have gluten, which means baked goods stick more. Be sure your pans and cookie sheets are greased especially well. Avoid sprays, since these often contain artificial ingredients. Just rub some plain ol' softened butter all over your pan or sheet. You can also use parchment paper or silicone baking mats. All your cookies, cakes, and more should come right off the sheet or out of the pan cleanly.

Chapter 3:

Keto desserts tips and faqs

The most frequent problems that many people have is that they don't plan ahead for situations where they know they are likely to get hungry before they can easily find access to another ketogenic meal. This type of situation is extremely easy to prepare for, especially if you already have some fat bombs on hand, or you can even experiment with premade keto options. The important thing is that you prevent yourself from getting so hungry that you are overly concerned with filling the hole in your stomach and not nearly concerned enough with filling your void with nutritious alternatives. Additionally, you will want to ensure that you try and eat at the same time each day to help your body learn when to expect its next meal. This will be especially important for when you exercise as you will want to eat some healthy fats beforehand to ensure you have the energy to give it your all. When you are finished, you will want to be sure to follow it up with protein to help your muscles get the most from the experience as possible. If you find yourself ending up too hungry after you exercise, keep in mind that a long, mild, workout is just as effective as a short, intense, workout and much less demanding on the body. Stretch things out, and you will likely find that you have less of an urge to binge after you are finished.

Shirataki noodles are your friend: While you might not have heard of the shirataki noodle yet, if you plan on sticking to the keto diet for a prolonged period of time it will soon be your best friend. Also known as the miracle noodle, shirataki noodles are made from the konjac plant and then formed into either noodles or rice. Shirataki noodles have one net gram of carbs per 100 grams of noodles which is far more than you will consume in an average serving. While they aren't nutritious, they are a good source of fiber and is a great way to make a wide variety of non-keto dishes keto without having to change anything else about them.

In addition to this major benefit, studies show that the type of fiber found in the shirataki noodle, known as glucomannan, has numerous different benefits on its own. First, it is proven to decrease feelings of hunger more effectively than other types of fiber which means that eating it as part of a meal will naturally make it easier for you to eat healthy portion sizes. Additionally, it is known to decrease several of the risk factors for heart disease including fasting blood sugar, cholesterol, triglycerides and LDL cholesterol. If you have issues with overeating, it will also help your body to only absorb an appropriate amount of the fat, protein and carbs that you consume.

It is not without potential issues to be aware of, however. First and foremost, as it is known to expand up to 50 times in water, it can cause digestive issues including mild diarrhea, gas and bloating in some people who eat it. It is also known to reduce the overall bioavailability of some oral medications and supplements which means you will want to speak a doctor before adding it as a regular part of your diet if you feel this may concern you. Additionally, this response only occurs in a small fraction of the population which means that it is definitely worth trying and seeing how you like it.

Know your exact net carb limit: While you will want to stick to 15 or less net carbs per day when first entering ketosis, this is just to save you the hassle of determining the exact amount of net carbs that your body can handle. The fact of the matter is that each person will have a different net carb limit, which can also change over time. To provide yourself with all the data you need to ensure that you have an accurate idea of just what is going on.

One of the most popular ways of doing so these days is through the use of the MyFitnessPal app which is one of the most popular calorie tracking apps around today, and with good reason. The base version is free, though some of the paid features are useful to those who are following the keto diet. The app also sets itself apart with the ease at which it is to share the progress. The app has a very large food database, but anyone can edit it, so it can sometimes be difficult to tell if the macros are reliable. Finally, the free version only tracks regular carbs, plus fiber so you will have to do a little math as well.

If you are looking for something that is tailored to the keto diet specifically, then you may be interested in Cronometer. While it costs

$2.99, it comes with an officially curated food database which provides far more details about the foods you are considering putting into your body in addition to natively calculating keto macros.

Being able to precisely track what you are eating comes with numerous benefits on its own as well. First and foremost, you will find that you can exert willpower over what you are eating much more easily when you know you have to account for it specifically. Additionally, it will help you to get a more accurate picture of what you are consuming during the day as you will be surprised at how many small things you eat during the day that you don't think of as either eating a meal or snacking. Finally, it will help to ensure that you get in the habit of measuring the foods you eat until you have an accurate idea of what a true serving size is. When done properly, watching your net carbs closely will make it possible to slowly ramp up the number of net carbs you can consume in a day without putting your ketogenic state at risk. While this may seem cumbersome and restrictive at first, it should be an easy habit to get into, and the end result will be more carbs, and thus more options, in your diet which will more than make up for the early hassle.

Be aware of ketoacidosis: Ketoacidosis is a deadly combination of overly high ketone levels, metabolic acidosis, and hyperglycemia that kills around 5,000 people per year, a vast majority of those are people who were already dealing with complications as a result of diabetes. If you are not one the roughly 400 million people worldwide who are dealing with some type of diabetes, then the odds of you contracting this condition are negligible. You would have to put yourself through the type of years of poor eating, lack of exercise and extreme stress that causes type 2 diabetes before your odds of contracting ketoacidosis began to increase. For those who are dealing with diabetes, the keto diet is still quite safe, as long as they are actively dealing with any issues that may cause them to end up with an untreated insulin deficiency. Ketoacidosis often occurs quite quickly, in as little as 24 hours. Symptoms include vomiting and abdominal pain, in addition to an increased heart rate, high blood glucose levels, and low blood pressure. The person suffering from ketoacidosis will also start off alert and slowly become more and more drowsy as the condition worsens.

Remaining in ketosis while eating out: While planning ahead is the easiest way to ensure that eating at a restaurant like a normal human being isn't an overly complicated disaster, sometimes the unexpected happens, and you will find yourself with no choice but to face a menu unprepared. Keep the following rules in mind, and you will be able to make it through with your ketones intact.

First and foremost, you will want to stick to the basics. If you are at a fast food restaurant, then you will want to avoid anything that is likely to have had sugar added to it, which admittedly will be most of the menu. Nevertheless, you should be able to power through with some type of non- breaded meat, either plain or with cheese. While you may think you will be able to get away with a salad, even non-fast food restaurants typically fill their salads with light, leafy greens and berries, all of which are quite high in carbs. If you will get a salad, ensure it includes plenty of meat and that any dressing only comes on the side.

In general, whatever you order you will want to ensure that it is free of sauces or dressings as it can be very difficult to determine with any degree of certainty what is actually in them. In general, you can trust fattier salad dressings, in moderation, such as blue cheese, Caesar, and ranch. Even better, if possible simply ask for a side of butter.

If you aren't sure about finding something on the menu that works for you, don't be afraid to try a special request. While lower-tier restaurants may not always be able to meet your needs, it certainly never hurts to try, after all, you are a paying customer. At the end of the day, if you aren't 100 percent sure about a given dish, it is better to go without as opposed to risking 20 or more net carbs on a single meal. While sometimes you will simply have no choice, generally it will be easier to skip a single meal than to work to get your body back into ketosis.

Sticking to the diet while traveling: While traveling can make remaining in a state of ketosis more challenging, once again it is more a matter of planning ahead than anything else. If you ever put off dealing with the food issue until the last minute, then you will have a more difficult time of it, guaranteed.

When traveling, the first thing you will want to do is to find a hotel that includes a kitchenette. This will make the entire process much more manageable, and with a quick trip to a local grocery store, you can have some of your favorites on hand at all times to ensure you aren't tempted into doing something that you will regret later on. The best part is that these types of special accommodations rarely cost much more than a more traditional room would as well. Just make sure you call ahead and ensure you have everything that you require from a kitchenette, as what qualifies can vary by location.

Beyond that, planning for your daily meals shouldn't be all that more difficult than when you plan for such things at home. All it really takes is a little legwork on a popular search engine as wherever you go there is likely an active keto community that can tell you all of the best restaurants and dishes to try regardless of your personal preferences. The biggest thing to keep in mind here is not to let the fact that you are on vacation justify eating poorly. While it might be a thrill to eat a week's worth of carbs in a day, you will most certainly regret it in the morning. Don't make that mistake, stay strong, you will be glad you did in the long run.

Eating keto on the cheap: While switching to a keto diet will likely leave you feeling better than you have in years, it can also be costlier, simply because of the fact that foods that are loaded with carbs are also often cheaper than the alternative. Luckily, it is perfectly possible to remain keto without breaking the bank. To get started, the first thing you will want to do is shop normally for a month or so to get a feel for the types of products you are most likely going to want to see more of.

While niche markets such as Whole Foods and Traders Joes will offer up plenty of products targeted at your demographic, if you are looking to save money then you will want to avoid these places like the plague. For starters, you will want to get a membership to a big box store like Costco or Sam's Club. These places routinely sell large cuts of meat for pennies on the dollar. What you don't use right away you can store, just be sure to go through the proper steps and use some type of vacuum sealer for the best results. You will also want to be sure that you mark everything with the date that you stored it to ensure that you rotate your stock regularly. Additionally, when shopping you will want to focus on the core components of your meals, not purchasing pre-made meals, regardless of whether they are keto or not. The cost of buying a pre- made meal is often at least a third higher than buying all of the ingredients separately. While you will almost certainly need more time to eat keto, the results are more than worth it.

Here are some tips if you mess up with your keto diet and ways to get back into a low-carb diet.

- Take notes: It's very common for keto to go off the rails and eat sugar or carbs. It might be fun in the beginning, but then the next day, you will feel serious discomfort and physically unwell like headache, stomach ache and inflammation. Moreover, it's quite easy to forget what you eat. Therefore, you need to remember your food and what you feel, and the best way is to write it down. So, make a habit of writing regularly about what you eat and how you feel about it. This could create a great significance in the future for you.

- Go for intermittent fasting: Intermittent fasting is widely recognized health practice in a Ketogenic diet. It's an opportunity for your body to deal with its toxic and junk you have eaten and detox it. Therefore, eat only when you feel really hungry and make sure that you next mean is Keto and don't forget to enjoy and savor it.

- Go Physical: You will fell a little low when you begin with exercise on a Ketogenic diet. It might hurt in the beginning, but afterward, you will feel much better. This doesn't mean that you have to do some high-intensity exercise. Just do some light exercise that raises your heartbeat for at least 15 minutes and breaks a sweat. A little exercise will clear your mind, improve digestion and control insulin level in the body.

- Sip water more: Being on Keto means that your body will lose lots of water. Although it is suggested to drink electrolyte drinks to provide your body with critical salts and keep it hydrated. What works more is simply drinking a cool liquid to make you feel energetic and on track.

  You can help yourself with herbal teas, without sweetener as well or something more flavorful to tickle your taste buds. Sip some warm bone broth; it will not fill your tummy without getting any carbs in it; it is satisfying and comforting as well.

- Sleep more: When your body switches to fats for energy, you could start losing your sleep as well. But you need to get a proper amount of sleep. Not getting enough sleep can disturb your Ketogenic lifestyle as it will prevent your body from functioning as it should be. Moreover, if you sleep enough, you are also preparing your body to handle the changes that come with implementing a Ketogenic lifestyle.

- Find a support group: Motivation is an essential factor to stay on the course. You need to promise yourself that you will follow the Ketogenic lifestyle with dedication. However, that promise you made in person can be easily broken. To avoid this, say it out loud in front of a support group or friends, you will feel that it's not easy to break. Therefore, find this support, you are numerous groups and forums online, and people there are very helpful and supportive, and they will also give you more ideas to help to keep you on track.

- Search some fun recipes: Another way to keep yourself excited is to turn the cooking and to eat Keto food into a fun activity. There are a number of websites and blogs with a lot of high-fat dessert recipes that are wonderful to make and satisfy your hunger.

In the following chapter, I have gathered some mouthwatering decadent desserts, from brownies, mousse, pies and frozen desserts, which will take your taste buds to gastronomical heaven. So, go into your kitchen and cook up some of your favorite desserts. Our Keto desserts incorporate a variety of Keto-friendly sugar substitutes. These sweeteners produce a sweet taste that is very close to sugar, but neither of these sweeteners converts into glucose or disturb ketosis. With all these tempting prospects, you should bear one thing in mind: just because the sweeteners are Keto friendly and have no calorie content, it doesn't mean that they can be consumed without limits. So, the best thumb rule is just to have sweet enough to tame your cravings.

Frequent Questions

Question #1: Who should avoid the Keto diet techniques? Before you make any decisions to begin the plan, consult your physician if you have suffered from any of the following:

- Impaired liver function
- History of pancreatitis
- Gallbladder related issues
- Gastric bypass surgery
- Impaired fat digestion
- History of kidney failure
- Women who are pregnant or lactating

At this point, you are making a meaningful change, and you should consult your personal dietitian or doctor for advice before moving forward.

Question#2: How can I make the process easier? Prepare a Menu and Food Plan: Use some of the recipes in this book and combine them with your other ketogenic favorites. You will be surprised how many tasty items you can enjoy that are full of healthy nutrients.

Question #3: Do I need to stop eating regularly? "Don't Try to Starve Yourself." Another major misconception of dieting is that you have to starve yourself to see results and that can actually be damaging your long-term health. This is just not true with the methods used on the ketogenic plan.

Question #4: Is the Keto Diet a restrictive diet that tastes bad? Don't Restrict Your Diet Severely: Diet foods don't have to taste bad. This is one of the most common misconceptions about diets – people think that diet foods have to taste bad. It's just not right! Explore your options and discover all the delicious meals you can make a daily part of your life.

Chapter 4:

Keto Desserts Recipes (50 Recipes)

Bars

Beginner

1. Pumpkin Bars

<u>Serves: 16</u>

<u>Preparation time: 10 minutes</u>

<u>Cooking time: 28 minutes</u>

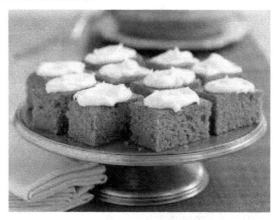

<u>Ingredients:</u>

- 2 eggs

- 1 ½ tsp pumpkin pie spice
- ½ tsp baking soda
- 1 tsp baking powder
- ¼ cup coconut flour
- 8 oz pumpkin puree
- ½ cup coconut oil, melted
- 1/3 cup Swerve
- Pinch of salt

Directions:

- Preheat the oven to 350 F/ 180 C.
- Spray 9*9 inch baking pan with cooking spray and set aside.
- In a bowl, beat eggs, sweetener, coconut oil, pumpkin pie spice, and pumpkin puree until well combined.
- In another bowl, mix together coconut flour, baking soda, baking powder, and salt.
- Add coconut flour mixture to the egg mixture and mix well.
- Pour bar mixture into the prepared baking pan and spread evenly.
- Bake in preheated oven for 28 minutes.
- Allow to cool completely then slice and serve.

Per Serving: Net Carbs: 1.1g; Calories: 73; Total Fat: 7.5g; Saturated Fat: 6.1g Protein: 0.9g; Carbs: 1.6g; Fiber: 0.5g; Sugar: 0.5g; Fat 90% / Protein 4% / Carbs 6%

2. Flavors Pumpkin Bars

<u>**Serves: 18**</u>

<u>**Preparation time: 10 minutes**</u>

<u>**Cooking time: 10 minutes**</u>

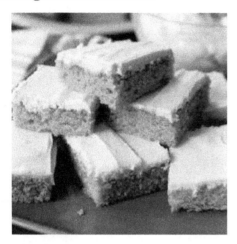

Ingredients:

- 1 tbsp coconut flour

- ½ tsp cinnamon

- 2 tsp pumpkin pie spice

- 1 tsp liquid stevia

- ½ cup erythritol

- 15 oz can pumpkin puree

- 15 oz can unsweetened coconut milk

- 16 oz cocoa butter

Directions:

- Line baking dish with parchment paper and set aside.

- Melt cocoa butter in a small saucepan over low heat.

- Add pumpkin puree and coconut milk and stir well.

- Add remaining ingredients and whisk well.

- Stir the mixture continuously until mixture thickens.

- Once the mixture thickens then pour it into prepared baking dish and place in the refrigerator for 2 hours.

- Slice and serve.

Per Serving: Net Carbs: 5.8g; Calories: 282; Total Fat: 28.1g; Saturated Fat: 17.1g Protein: 1.3g; Carbs: 9.5g; Fiber: 3.7g; Sugar: 4g; Fat 89% / Protein 2% / Carbs 9%

3. Coconut Lemon Bars

<u>**Serves: 24**</u>

<u>**Preparation time: 10 minutes**</u>

<u>**Cooking time: 42 minutes**</u>

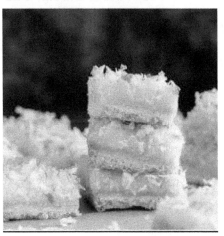

<u>**Ingredients:**</u>

- 4 eggs

- 1 tbsp coconut flour

- 3/4 cup Swerve

- 1/2 tsp baking powder

- 1/3 cup fresh lemon juice

- For crust:

- 1/4 cup Swerve

- 2 1/4 cups almond flour

- 1/2 cup coconut oil, melted

Directions:

- Preheat the oven to 350 F/ 180 C.

- Spray a baking dish with cooking spray and set aside.

- In a small bowl, mix together 1/4 cup swerve and almond flour.

- Add melted coconut oil and mix until it forms into a dough.

- Transfer dough into the prepared pan and spread evenly.

- Bake for 15 minutes.

- For the filling: Add eggs, coconut flour, baking powder, lemon juice, and swerve into the blender and blend for 10 seconds.

- Pour blended mixture on top of baked crust and spread well.

- Bake for 25 minutes.

- Remove from oven and set aside to cool completely.

- Slice and serve.

Per Serving: Net Carbs: 1.5g; Calories: 113; Total Fat: 10.6g; Saturated Fat: 4.6g Protein: 3.3g; Carbs: 2.8g; Fiber: 1.3g; Sugar: 0.5g; Fat 84% / Protein 11% / Carbs 5%

4. Protein Bars

Serves: 8

Preparation time: 10 minutes

Cooking time: 10 minutes

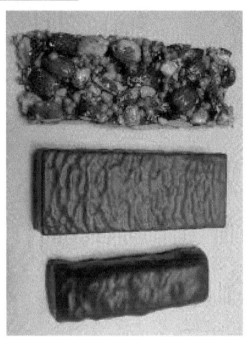

Ingredients:

- 2 scoops vanilla protein powder

- ½ tsp cinnamon

- 15 drops liquid stevia

- ¼ cup coconut oil, melted

- 1 cup almond butter

- Pinch of salt

Directions:

- In a bowl, mix together all ingredients until well combined.

- Transfer bar mixture into a baking dish and press down evenly.

- Place in refrigerator until firm.

- Slice and serve.

Per Serving: Net Carbs: 0.2g; Calories: 99 Total Fat: 8g; Saturated Fat: 6g Protein: 7.2g; Carbs: 0.6g; Fiber: 0.4g; Sugar: 0.2g; Fat 71% / Protein 28% / Carbs 1%

5. Easy Lemon Bars

<u>Serves: 8</u>

<u>Preparation time: 10 minutes</u>

<u>Cooking time: 40 minutes</u>

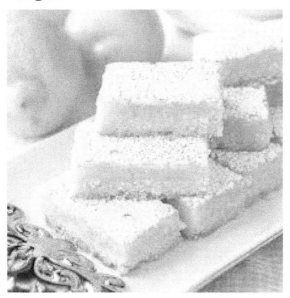

<u>Ingredients:</u>

- 4 eggs

- 1/3 cup erythritol

- 2 tsp baking powder

- 2 cups almond flour

- 1 lemon zest

- ¼ cup fresh lemon juice

- ½ cup butter softened

- ½ cup sour cream

Directions:

- Preheat the oven to 350 F/ 180 C.

- Line 9*6-inch baking pan with parchment paper. Set aside.

- In a bowl, beat eggs until frothy.

- Add butter and sour cream and beat until well combined.

- Add sweetener, lemon zest, and lemon juice and blend well.

- Add baking powder and almond flour and mix until well combined.

- Transfer batter in a prepared baking pan and spread evenly.

- Bake in preheated oven for 35-40 minutes.

- Remove from oven and allow to cool completely.

- Slice and serve.

Per Serving: Net Carbs: 4.9g; Calories: 329; Total Fat: 30.8g; Saturated Fat: 10.9g Protein: 9.5g; Carbs: 8.2g; Fiber: 3.3g; Sugar: 1.5g; Fat 84% / Protein 11% / Carbs 5%

Intermediate

6. Peanut Butter Bars

<u>**Serves: 9**</u>

<u>**Preparation time: 10 minutes**</u>

<u>**Cooking time: 30 minutes**</u>

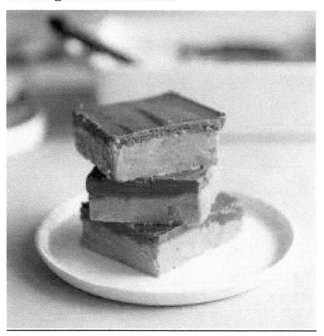

<u>**Ingredients:**</u>

- 2 eggs

- 1 tbsp coconut flour

- ¼ cup almond flour

- ½ cup erythritol

- ½ cup butter softened

- ½ cup peanut butter

Keto desserts for Beginners

Directions:

- Spray 9*9-inch baking pan with cooking spray and set aside.

- In a bowl, beat together butter, eggs, and peanut butter until well combined.

- Add dry ingredients and mix until a smooth batter is formed.

- Spread batter evenly in prepared baking pan.

- Bake at 350 F/ 180 C for 30 minutes.

- Slice and serve.

Per Serving: Net Carbs: 2.8g; Calories: 213; Total Fat: 20.2g; Saturated Fat: 8.6g Protein: 5.8g; Carbs: 4.5g; Fiber: 1.7g; Sugar: 1.7g; Fat 85% / Protein 10% / Carbs 5%

7.Saffron Coconut Bars

<u>**Serves: 15**</u>

<u>**Preparation time: 10 minutes**</u>

<u>**Cooking time: 15**</u>

<u>**minutes**</u>

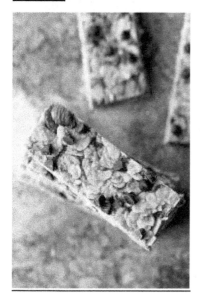

<u>Ingredients:</u>

- 1 3/4 cups unsweetened shredded coconut

- 8 saffron threads

- 1 1/3 cups unsweetened coconut milk

- 1 tsp cardamom powder

- 1/4 cup Swerve

- 3.5 oz ghee

<u>Directions:</u>

- Spray a square baking dish with cooking spray and set aside.

- In a bowl, mix together coconut milk and shredded coconut and set aside for half an hour.

- Add sweetener and saffron and mix well to combine.

- Melt ghee in a pan over medium heat.

- Add coconut mixture to the pan and cook for 5-7 minutes.

- Add cardamom powder and cook for 3-5 minutes more.

- Transfer coconut mixture into the prepared baking dish and spread evenly.

- Place in refrigerator for 1-2 hours.

- Slice and serve.

Per Serving: Net Carbs: 1.7g; Calories: 191 Total Fat: 19.2g; Saturated Fat: 15.1g Protein: 1.5g; Carbs: 4.1g; Fiber: 2.4g; Sugar: 1.6g; Fat 91% / Protein 5% / Carbs 4%

8. Cheese Chocolate Bars

<u>**Serves: 16**</u>

<u>**Preparation time: 10 minutes**</u>

<u>**Cooking time: 10 minutes**</u>

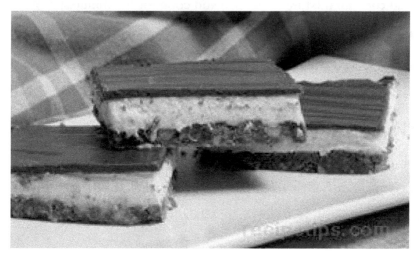

<u>Ingredients:</u>

- 16 oz cream cheese, softened

- 14 oz unsweetened dark chocolate

- 1 tsp vanilla

- 12 drops liquid stevia

<u>Directions:</u>

- Spray 8-inch square pan with cooking spray and set aside.

- Melt chocolate in a saucepan over low heat.

- Stir in sweetener and vanilla. Remove from heat and set aside.

- Add cream cheese into the food processor and process until smooth.

- Add melted chocolate mixture into the cream cheese and process until well combined.

- Transfer cheese chocolate mixture into the prepared pan and spread evenly.

- Place in refrigerator for 4 hours.

- Slice and serve.

Per Serving: Net Carbs: 4.1g; Calories: 265; Total Fat: 23.1g; Saturated Fat: 14.5g Protein: 5.5g; Carbs: 7.4g; Fiber: 3.3g; Sugar: 0.1g; Fat 82% / Protein 11% / Carbs 7%

9. Coconut Bars

<u>__Serves: 24__</u>

<u>__Preparation time: 10 minutes__</u>

<u>__Cooking time: 10 minutes__</u>

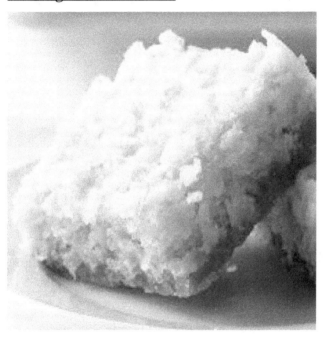

Ingredients:

- ¼ cup of coconut oil

- ½ cup erythritol

- 1/2 cup coconut cream

- 3 cups unsweetened desiccated coconut

Directions:

- Line 8*5-inch baking pan with parchment paper and set aside.

- Add all ingredients into the blender and blend until sticky mixture form.

- Transfer coconut mixture in prepared baking pan.

- Spread mixture evenly and press down with your hands.

- Place in refrigerator for 15 minutes.

- Slice and serve.

Per Serving: Net Carbs: 0.2g; Calories: 111; Total Fat: 12g; Saturated Fat: 6g Protein: 0.1g; Carbs: 0.3g; Fiber: 0.1g; Sugar: 0.2g; Fat 98% / Protein 1% / Carbs 1%

Expert

10.   **Butter Fudge Bars**

<u>**Serves: 36**</u>

<u>**Preparation time: 10**</u>

<u>**minutes**</u>

<u>**Cooking time: 10**</u>

<u>**minutes**</u>

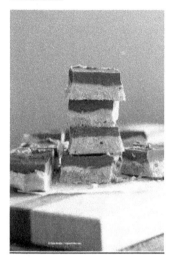

<u>Ingredients:</u>

- 1 cup unsweetened peanut butter

- 1/2 cup whey protein powder

- 1 tsp stevia

- 1 cup erythritol

- 8 oz cream cheese

- 1 tsp vanilla

- 1 cup butter

Directions:

- Spray baking pan with cooking spray and line with parchment paper. Set aside.

- Melt butter and cream cheese in a saucepan over medium heat.

- Add peanut butter and stir to combine.

- Remove pan from heat.

- Add remaining ingredients and blend until well combined.

- Pour mixture into the prepared pan and spread evenly.

- Place in refrigerator for 1-2 hours or until set.

- Slice and serve.

Per Serving: Net Carbs: 1.2g; Calories: 111; Total Fat: 11g; Saturated Fat: 5.3g Protein: 2.3g; Carbs: 1.6g; Fiber: 0.4g; Sugar: 0.5g; Fat 88% / Protein 8% / Carbs 4%

11.　Sesame Bars

<u>**Serves: 16**</u>

<u>**Preparation time: 10 minutes**</u>

<u>**Cooking time: 15 minutes**</u>

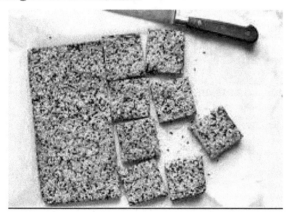

<u>Ingredients:</u>

- 1 1/4 cups sesame seeds

- 10 drops liquid stevia

- 1/2 tsp vanilla

- 1/4 cup unsweetened applesauce

- 3/4 cup coconut butter

- Pinch of salt

<u>Directions:</u>

- Preheat the oven to 350 F/ 180 C.

- Spray a baking dish with cooking spray and set aside.

- In a large bowl, add applesauce, coconut butter, vanilla, liquid stevia, and sea salt and stir until well combined.

- Add sesame seeds and stir to coat.

- Pour mixture into a prepared baking dish and bake in preheated oven for 10-15 minutes.

- Remove from oven and set aside to cool completely.

- Place in refrigerator for 1 hour.

- Cut into pieces and serve.

Per Serving: Net Carbs: 2.4g; Calories: 136 Total Fat: 12.4g; Saturated Fat: 6.8g Protein: 2.8g; Carbs: 5.7g; Fiber: 3.3g; Sugar: 1.2g; Fat 83% / Protein 9% / Carbs 8%

12.   Chocó Chip Bars

<u>**Serves: 24**</u>

<u>**Preparation time: 10 minutes**</u>

<u>**Cooking time: 35 minutes**</u>

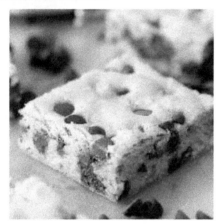

Ingredients:

- 1 cup walnuts, chopped

- 1 ½ tsp baking powder

- 1 cup unsweetened

- chocolate chips

- 1 cup almond flour

- ¼ cup coconut flour

- 1 ½ tsp vanilla

- 5 eggs

- ½ cup butter

- 8 oz cream cheese

- 2 cups erythritol

- Pinch of salt

Directions:

- 350 F/ 180 C should be the target when preheating oven.

- Line cookie sheet with parchment paper and set aside.

- Beat together butter, sweetener, vanilla, and cream cheese until smooth.

- Add eggs and beat until well combined.

- Add remaining ingredients and stir gently to combine.

- The mixture should be transferred to the prepared cookie sheet and spread evenly.

- Bake in preheated oven for 35 minutes.

- Remove from oven and allow to cool completely.

- Slice and serve.

Per Serving: Net Carbs: 2.6g; Calories: 207 Total Fat: 18.8 g; Saturated Fat: 8.5g Protein: 5.5g; Carbs: 4.8g; Fiber: 2.2g; Sugar: 0.4g; Fat 83% / Protein 11% / Carbs 6%

13. Coconut Peanut Butter Bars

Serves: 12

Preparation time: 10 minutes

Cooking time: 10 minutes

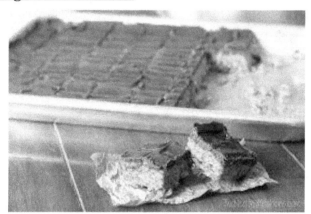

Ingredients:

- 1 cup unsweetened
- shredded coconut
- ½ tsp vanilla
- 1 tbsp swerve
- 1 cup creamy peanut butter
- ¼ cup butter
- Pinch of salt

Directions:

- Add butter in microwave safe bowl and microwave until butter is melted.

- Add peanut butter and stir well.

- Add sweetener, vanilla, and salt and stir.

- Add shredded coconut and mix until well combined.

- Transfer mixture into the greased baking dish and spread evenly.

- Place in refrigerator for 1 hour.

- Slice and serve.

Per Serving: Net Carbs: 3.8g; Calories: 221 Total Fat: 20g; Saturated Fat: 9.4g Protein: 6.1g; Carbs: 6.4g; Fiber: 2.6g; Sugar: 2.7g; Fat 82% / Protein 12% / Carbs 6

14.　**Blueberry Bars**

<u>**Serves: 4**</u>

<u>**Preparation time: 10 minutes**</u>

<u>**Cooking time: 75 minutes**</u>

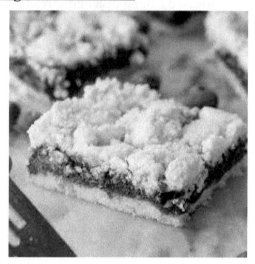

<u>**Ingredients:**</u>

- ¼ cup blueberries

- 1 tsp vanilla

- 1 tsp fresh lemon juice

- 2 tbsp erythritol

- ¼ cup almonds, sliced

- ¼ cup coconut flakes

- 3 tbsp coconut oil

- 2 tbsp coconut flour

- ½ cup almond flour

- 3 tbsp water

- 1 tbsp chia seeds

Directions:

- Preheat the oven to 300 F/ 150 C.

- Line baking dish with parchment paper and set aside.

- In a small bowl, mix together water and chia seeds. Set aside.

- In a bowl, combine together all ingredients. Add chia mixture and stir well.

- Pour mixture into the prepared baking dish and spread evenly.

- Bake for 50 minutes. Remove from oven and allow to cool completely.

- Cut into bars and serve.

Per Serving: Net Carbs: 2.8g; Calories: 136; Total Fat: 11.9g; Saturated Fat: 6.1g Protein: 3.1g; Carbs: 5.5g; Fiber: 2.7g; Sugar: 1.3g; Fat 81% / Protein 10% / Carbs 9%

Cake

Beginner

15.　Delicious Ricotta Cake

<u>**Serves: 8**</u>

<u>**Preparation time: 10 minutes**</u>

<u>**Cooking time: 45 minutes**</u>

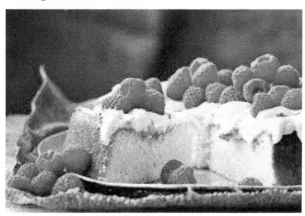

<u>**Ingredients:**</u>

- 2 eggs

- ½ cup erythritol

- ¼ cup coconut flour

- 15 oz ricotta

- Pinch of salt

<u>**Directions:**</u>

- Preheat the oven to 350 F/ 180 C.

- Spray 9-inch baking pan with cooking spray and set aside.

- In a bowl whisk eggs.

- Add remaining ingredients and mix until well combined.

- Transfer batter in prepared baking pan.

- Bake in preheated oven for 45 minutes.

- Remove baking pan from oven and allow to cool completely.

- Slice and serve.

Per Serving: Net Carbs: 2.9g; Calories: 91; Total Fat: 5.4g; Saturated Fat: 3g Protein: 7.5g; Carbs: 3.1g; Fiber: 0.2g; Sugar: 0.3g; Fat 55% / Protein 33% / Carbs 12%

16.   Chocó Coconut Cake

<u>**Serves: 9**</u>

<u>**Preparation time: 10 minutes**</u>

<u>**Cooking time: 25 minutes**</u>

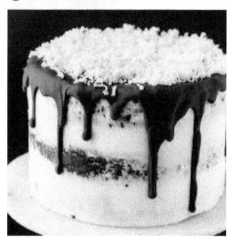

<u>Ingredients:</u>

- 6 eggs

- 1 tsp vanilla

- 3 oz butter, melted

- 11.5 oz heavy whipping cream

- 2 tsp baking powder

- 3 oz unsweetened cocoa powder

- 5 oz erythritol

- 3.5 oz coconut flour

<u>Directions:</u>

- Preheat the oven to 350 F/ 180 C.

- In a bowl, mix together coconut flour, butter, 5.5 oz heavy whipping cream, eggs, baking powder 1.5 oz cocoa powder, and 3 oz erythritol until well combined.

- Pour batter into the greased cake pan and bake in preheated oven for 25 minutes.

- Remove cake from oven and allow to cool completely.

- In a large bowl, beat remaining heavy whipping cream, cocoa powder, and erythritol until smooth.

- Spread the cream on the cake evenly.

- Place cake in the refrigerator for 30 minutes.

- Slice and serve.

Per Serving: Net Carbs: 5g; Calories: 282 Total Fat: 26.1g; Saturated Fat: 15.6g Protein: 7.1g; Carbs: 10.1g; Fiber: 5.1g; Sugar: 0.9g; Fat 83% / Protein 10% / Carbs 7%

17.   Fudgy Chocolate Cake

Serves: 12

Preparation time: 10 minutes

Cooking time: 30 minutes

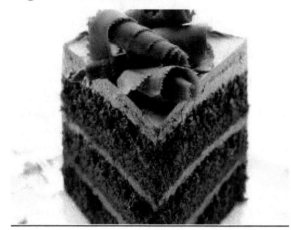

Ingredients:

- 6 eggs

- 1 ½ cup erythritol

- ½ cup almond flour

- 10.5 oz butter, melted

- 10.5 oz unsweetened chocolate, melted

- Pinch of salt

Directions:

- Preheat the oven to 350 F/ 180 C.

- Grease 8-inch spring-form cake pan with butter and set aside.

- In a large bowl, beat eggs until foamy.

- Add sweetener and stir well.

- Add melted butter, chocolate, almond flour, and salt and stir until combined.

- Pour batter in the prepared cake pan and bake in preheated oven for 30 minutes.

- Remove cake from oven and allow to cool completely.

- Slice and serve.

Per Serving: Net Carbs: 4g; Calories: 360; Total Fat: 37.6g; Saturated Fat: 21.6g Protein: 7.2g; Carbs: 8.6g; Fiber: 4.6g; Sugar: 0.6g; Fat 90% / Protein 7% / Carbs 3%

18.   Cinnamon Almond Cake

Serves: 6

Preparation time: 10 minutes

Cooking time: 20 minutes

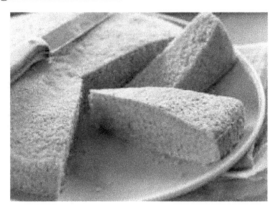

Ingredients:

- 4 eggs

- 1 tsp orange zest

- 2/3 cup dried cranberries

- 1 ½ cups almond flour

- 1 tsp vanilla extract

- 2 tsp mixed spice

- 2 tsp cinnamon

- ¼ cup erythritol

- 1 cup butter, softened

Directions:

- Preheat the oven to 350 F/ 180 C.

- In a bowl, add sweetener and melted butter and beat until fluffy.

- Add cinnamon, vanilla, and mixed spice and stir well.

- Add egg one by one and stir until well combined.

- Add almond flour, orange zest, and cranberries and mix until well combined.

- Pour batter in a greased cake pan and bake in preheated oven for 20 minutes.

- Slice and serve.

Per Serving: Net Carbs: 4.3g; Calories: 484; Total Fat: 47.6g; Saturated Fat: 21.3g Protein: 10g; Carbs: 8.2g; Fiber: 3.9g; Sugar: 1.8g; Fat 88% / Protein 8% / Carbs 4%

Intermediate

19.   Lemon Cake

<u>**Serves: 10**</u>

<u>**Preparation time: 10 minutes**</u>

<u>**Cooking time: 60 minutes**</u>

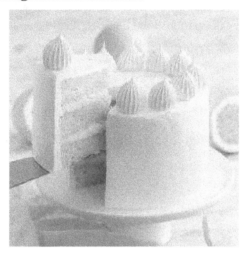

<u>**Ingredients:**</u>

- 4 eggs

- 2 tbsp lemon zest

- ½ cup fresh lemon juice

- ¼ cup erythritol

- 1 tbsp vanilla

- ½ cup butter softened

- 2 tsp baking powder

- ¼ cup coconut flour

- 2 cups almond flour

Directions:

- Preheat the oven to 300 F/ 150 C.

- Grease 9-inch loaf pan with butter and set aside.

- In a large bowl, whisk all ingredients until a smooth batter is formed.

- Pour batter into the loaf pan and bake in preheated oven for 60 minutes.

- Slice and serve.

Per Serving: Net Carbs: 3.6g; Calories: 244; Total Fat: 22.3g; Saturated Fat: 7.3g Protein: 7.3g; Carbs: 6.3g; Fiber: 2.7g; Sugar: 1.5g; Fat 83% / Protein 12% / Carbs 5%

20.   Vanilla Butter Cake

<u>**Serves: 9**</u>

<u>**Preparation time: 10 minutes**</u>

<u>**Cooking time: 35 minutes**</u>

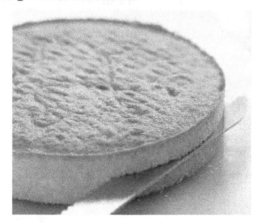

<u>**Ingredients:**</u>

- 5 eggs

- 1 tsp baking powder

- oz almond flour

- 1/2 cup butter, softened

- 1 cup Swerve

- 4 oz cream cheese, softened

- 1 tsp vanilla

- 1 tsp orange extract

<u>**Directions:**</u>

- Preheat the oven to 350 F/ 180 C.

- Spray 9-inch cake pan with cooking spray and set aside.

- Add all ingredients into the mixing bowl and whisk until batter is fluffy.

- Pour batter into the prepared pan and bake in preheated oven for 35-40 minutes.

- Remove cake from oven and set aside to cool completely.

- Slices and serve.

Per Serving: Net Carbs: 3.3g; Calories: 289; Total Fat: 27.2g; Saturated Fat: 10.7g Protein: 8.5g; Carbs: 5.5g; Fiber: 2.2g; Sugar: 1.1g; Fat 85% / Protein 11% / Carbs 4%

21. Carrot Cake

Serves: 16

Preparation time: 10 minutes

Cooking time: 35 minutes

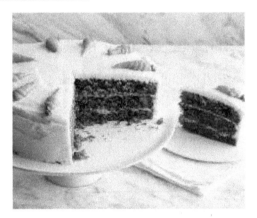

Ingredients:

- 2 eggs

- ½ tsp vanilla

- 2 tbsp butter, melted

- ½ cup carrots, grated

- 1/8 tsp ground cloves

- 1 tsp cinnamon

- 1 tsp baking powder

- 2 tbsp unsweetened shredded coconut

- ¼ cup pecans, chopped

- 6 tbsp erythritol

- ¾ cup almond flour

- Pinch of salt

Directions:

- Preheat the oven to 325 F/ 162 C.

- Spray cake pan with cooking spray and set aside.

- In a large bowl, whisk together almond flour, cloves, cinnamon, baking powder, shredded coconut, nuts, sweetener, and salt.

- Stir in eggs, vanilla, butter, and shredded coconut until well combined.

- Pour batter into the prepared cake pan and bake in preheated oven for 30-35 minutes.

- Slice and serve.

Per Serving: Net Carbs: 1.4g; Calories: 111 Total Fat: 10.6g; Saturated Fat: 2.2g Protein: 2.7g; Carbs: 3g; Fiber: 1.6g; Sugar: 0.7g; Fat 86% / Protein 9% / Carbs 5%

22.   Delicious Almond Cake

<u>**Serves: 16**</u>

<u>**Preparation time: 10 minutes**</u>

<u>**Cooking time: 40 minutes**</u>

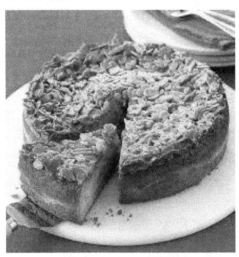

<u>**Ingredients:**</u>

- 4 eggs

- 1 tsp baking powder

- 1 1/2 tsp vanilla

- 1/3 cup Swerve

- 2 oz cream cheese, softened

- 2 tbsp butter

- 1 cup almond flour

- 1/2 cup coconut flour

- 4 oz half and half

- Pinch of salt

- For topping:

- 3/4 cup almonds, toasted and sliced

- 1/3 cup Swerve

- 6 tbsp butter, melted

- 1 cup almond flour

Directions:

- Preheat the oven to 350 F/ 180 C.

- Spray 8-inch cake pan with cooking spray and set aside.

- Add all ingredients except topping ingredients into the large bowl whisk until well combined.

- Pour batter into the prepared cake pan and spread evenly.

- Combine together all topping ingredients.

- Sprinkle topping mixture evenly on top of batter.

- Bake for 40 minutes.

- Remove from oven and allow to cool completely.

- Slice and serve.

Per Serving: Net Carbs: 2.8g; Calories: 198 Total Fat: 18.2g; Saturated Fat: 6g Protein: 5.9g; Carbs: 5g; Fiber: 2.2g; Sugar: 0.9g; Fat 83% / Protein 12% / Carbs 5%

Expert

23.　Lemon Cheesecake

<u>Serves: 8</u>

<u>Preparation time: 10 minutes</u>

<u>Cooking time: 55 minutes</u>

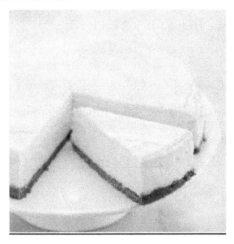

Ingredients:

- 4 eggs

- 18 oz ricotta cheese

- 1 fresh lemon zest

- 2 tbsp swerve

- 1 fresh lemon juice

Directions:

- Preheat the oven to 350 F/ 180 C.

- Spray cake pan with cooking spray and set aside.

- In a large bowl, beat ricotta cheese until smooth.

- Add egg one by one and whisk well.

- Add lemon juice, lemon zest, and swerve and mix well.

- Transfer mixture into the prepared cake pan and bake for 50-55 minutes.

- Remove cake from oven and set aside to cool completely.

- Place cake in the fridge for 1-2 hours.

- Slice and serve.

Per Serving: Net Carbs: 4.6g; Calories: 124; Total Fat: 7.3g; Saturated Fat: 3.9g Protein: 10.2g; Carbs: 4.8g; Fiber: 0.2g; Sugar: 0.7g; Fat 53% / Protein 33% / Carbs 14%

24.   Delicious Cheesecake

Serves: 8

Preparation time: 15 minutes

Cooking time: 1 hour 20 minutes

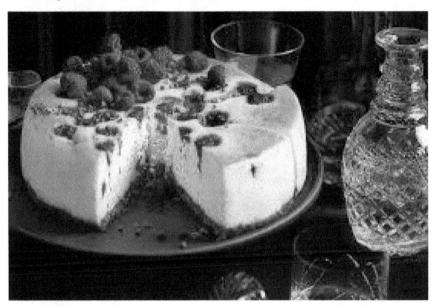

Ingredients:

- 3 eggs

- 1/4 cup shredded coconut

- 1/2 cup coconut flour

- 1/2 cup almond flour

- 1 tsp vanilla

- 1 tbsp stevia

- 15.5 oz sour cream

- 8 oz cream cheese, softened

- 1/2 cup butter, melted

Directions:

- Preheat the oven 300 F/ 150 C.

- Spray 9-inch spring-form pan with cooking spray. Set aside.

- For the crust: In a mixing bowl, mix together coconut flour, almond flour, shredded coconut, and melted butter until well combined.

- Transfer crust mixture into the prepared pan and spread evenly and press down with a fingertip.

- Place pan into the fridge to set crust.

- For the cheesecake filling: In a large bowl, beat sour cream and cream cheese together.

- Add egg, vanilla, and sweetener and beat until well combined.

- Pour cheesecake filling evenly over crust.

- Place pan in a water bath and bake for 1 hour-1 hour 20 minutes.

- Remove cake pan from oven and set aside to cool completely.

- Place cake pan into the fridge for 5-6 hours.

- Slice and serve.

Per Serving: Net Carbs: 5.9g; Calories: 400; Total Fat: 39g; Saturated Fat: 22.3g Protein: 7.8g; Carbs: 7.2g; Fiber: 1.3g; Sugar: 2.3g; Fat 86% / Protein 8% / Carbs 6%

25. Pumpkin Cheesecake

Serves: 8

Preparation time: 15 minutes

Cooking time: 1 hour 10 minutes

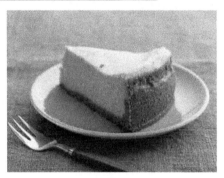

Ingredients:

For Crust:

- 1/2 cup almond flour

- 1 tbsp swerve

- 1/4 cup butter, melted

- 1 tbsp flaxseed meal

  For Filling:

- 3 eggs

- 1/2 tsp ground cinnamon

- 1/2 tsp vanilla

- 2/3 cup pumpkin puree

- 15.5 oz cream cheese

- 1/4 tsp ground nutmeg

- 2/3 cup Swerve

- Pinch of salt

Directions:

- Preheat the oven to 300 F/ 150 C.

- Spray 9-inch spring-form pan with cooking spray. Set aside.

- For Crust: In a bowl, mix together almond flour, swerve, flaxseed meal, and salt.

- Add melted butter and mix well to combine.

- Transfer crust mixture into the prepared pan and press down evenly with a fingertip.

- Bake for 10-15 minutes.

- Remove from oven and allow to cool for 10 minutes.

- For the cheesecake filling: In a large bowl, beat cream cheese until smooth and creamy.

- Add eggs, vanilla, swerve, pumpkin puree, nutmeg, cinnamon, and salt and stir until well combined.

- Pour cheesecake batter into the prepared crust and spread evenly.

- Bake for 50-55 minutes.

- Remove cheesecake from oven and set aside to cool completely.

- Place cheesecake in the fridge for 4 hours. Slices and serve.

Per Serving: Net Carbs: 3.9g; Calories: 320 Total Fat: 30.4g; Saturated Fat: 16.6g Protein: 8.2g; Carbs: 5.6g; Fiber: 1.7g; Sugar: 1.2g; Fat 86% / Protein 10% / Carbs 4%

26. Flourless Chocó Cake

Serves: 8

Preparation time: 10 minutes

Cooking time: 45 minutes

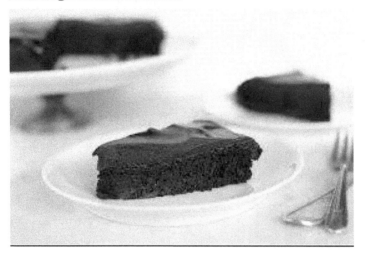

Ingredients:

- 7oz unsweetened dark chocolate,

- chopped

- ¼ cup Swerve

- 4 eggs, separated

- 3.5 oz cream

- 3.5 oz butter, cubed

Directions:

- Grease 8-inch cake pan with butter and set aside.

- Add butter and chocolate in microwave safe bowl and microwave until melted. Stir well.

- Add sweetener and cream and mix well.

- Add egg yolks one by one and mix until combined.

- In another bowl, beat egg whites until stiff peaks form.

- Gently fold egg whites into the chocolate mixture.

- Pour batter in the prepared cake pan and bake at 325 F/ 162 C for 45 minutes.

- Slice and serve.

Per Serving: Net Carbs: 5.1g; Calories: 318; Total Fat: 28.2g; Saturated Fat: 17g Protein: 6.6g; Carbs: 8.4g; Fiber: 3.3g; Sugar: 1.2g; Fat 82% / Protein 10% / Carbs 8%

27.   Gooey Chocolate Cake

Serves: 8

Preparation time: 10 minutes

Cooking time: 20 minutes

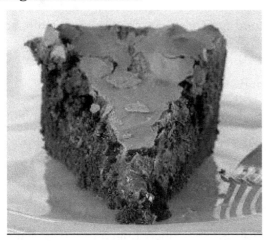

Ingredients:

- 2 eggs

- 1/4 cup unsweetened cocoa powder

- 1/2 cup almond flour

- 1/2 cup butter, melted

- 1 tsp vanilla

- 3/4 cup Swerve

- Pinch of salt

Directions:

- Preheat the oven to 350 F/ 180 C.

- Spray 8-inch spring-form cake pan with cooking spray. Set aside.

- In a bowl, sift together almond flour, cocoa powder, and salt. Mix well and set aside.

- In another bowl, whisk eggs, vanilla extract, and sweetener until creamy.

- Slowly fold the almond flour mixture into the egg mixture and stir well to combine.

- Add melted butter and stir well.

- Pour cake batter into the prepared pan and bake for 20 minutes.

- Remove from oven and allow to cool completely.

- Slice and serve.

Per Serving: Net Carbs: 1.7g; Calories: 166; Total Fat: 16.5g; Saturated Fat: 8.1g Protein: 3.5 g; Carbs: 3.3g; Fiber: 1.6g; Sugar: 0.5g; Fat 88% / Protein 8% / Carbs 4%

28. Coconut Cake

Serves: 8

Preparation time: 10 minutes

Cooking time: 20 minutes

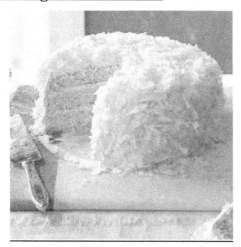

Ingredients:

- 5 eggs, separated

- ½ tsp baking powder

- ½ tsp vanilla

- ½ cup butter softened

- ½ cup erythritol

- ¼ cup unsweetened coconut milk

- ½ cup coconut flour

- Pinch of salt

Directions:

- Preheat the oven to 400 F/ 200 C.

- Grease cake pan with butter and set aside.

- In a bowl, beat sweetener and butter until combined.

- Add egg yolks, coconut milk, and vanilla and mix well.

- Add baking powder, coconut flour, and salt and stir well.

- In another bowl, beat egg whites until stiff peak forms.

- Gently fold egg whites into the cake mixture.

- Pour batter in a prepared cake pan and bake in preheated oven for 20 minutes.

- Slice and serve.

Per Serving: Net Carbs: 0.8g; Calories: 163 Total Fat: 16.2g; Saturated Fat: 9.9g Protein: 3.9g; Carbs: 1.3g; Fiber: 0.5g; Sugar: 0.6g; Fat 89% / Protein 9% / Carbs 2%

Tarts and Pie

Beginner

29.   Peanut Butter Pie

<u>Serves: 16</u>

<u>Preparation time: 15 minutes</u>

<u>Cooking time: 10 minutes</u>

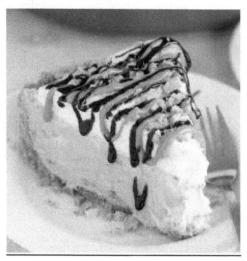

Ingredients:

For crust:

- ¾ cup almond flour

- ½ cup of cocoa powder

- ½ cup erythritol

- 1/3 cup almond butter

- ½ cup butter softened

For filling:

- 1 ½ cups heavy whipping cream

- ½ cup erythritol

- 1/3 cup peanut butter

- 8 oz cream cheese, softened

Directions:

For the crust:

- In a large bowl, combine together butter, cocoa powder, sweetener, and almond butter until smooth.

- Add almond flour and beat until mixture stiff.

- Transfer crust mixture into the greased spring-form cake pan and spread evenly and place in the refrigerator for 15-30 minutes.

- Meanwhile for filling: In a mixing bowl, beat sweetener, peanut butter, and cream cheese until smooth.

- Add heavy cream and beat until stiff peaks form.

- Spread filling mixture in prepared crust and refrigerate for 2 hours.

- Slice and serve.

Per Serving: Net Carbs: 2.7g; Calories: 209; Total Fat: 20.7g; Saturated Fat: 10.3g Protein: 4.4g; Carbs: 4.4g; Fiber: 1.7g; Sugar: 0.8g; Fat 88% / Protein 7% / Carbs 5%

30.   Delicious Blueberry Pie

<u>**Serves: 8**</u>

<u>**Preparation time: 10 minutes**</u>

<u>**Cooking time: 25 minutes**</u>

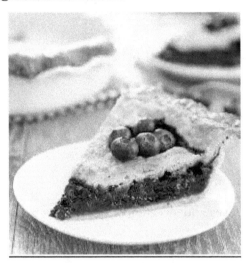

<u>**For crust:**</u>

- 4 eggs

- 1 tbsp water

- ¼ tsp baking powder

- 1 ½ cups coconut flour

- 1 cup butter, melted

- Pinch of salt

<u>**For filling:**</u>

- 8 oz cream cheese

- 2 tbsp swerve

- 1 ½ cup fresh blueberries

Directions:

- Spray 9-inch pie pan with cooking spray and set aside.

- In a large bowl, mix together all crust ingredients until dough is formed.

- Divide dough in half and roll out I between two parchment paper sheet and set aside.

- Preheat the oven to 350 F/ 180 C.

- Transfer one crust sheet into greased pie pan.

- Spread cream cheese on crust.

- Mix together blueberries and sweetener. Spread blueberries on top of the cream cheese layer.

- Cover pie with other half rolled crust and bake for 25 minutes.

- Allow to cool completely then slice and serve.

Per Serving: Net Carbs: 5.4g; Calories: 362 Total Fat: 35.6g; Saturated Fat: 21.9g Protein: 5.7g; Carbs: 7g; Fiber: 1.6g; Sugar: 3.1g; Fat 88% / Protein 6% / Carbs 6%

31. Quick & Simple Strawberry Tart

Serves: 10

Preparation time: 10 minutes

Cooking time: 22 minutes

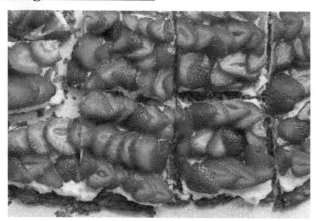

Ingredients:

- 5 egg whites

- ½ cup butter, melted

- 1 tsp baking powder

- 1 tsp vanilla

- 1 lemon zest, grated

- 1 ½ cup almond flour

- 1/3 cup xylitol

Directions:

- Preheat the oven to 375 F/ 190 C.

- Spray the tart pan with cooking spray and set aside.

- In a bowl, whisk egg whites until foamy.

- Add sweetener and whisk until soft peaks form.

- Add remaining ingredients except for strawberries and fold until well combined.

- Pour mixture into the prepared tart pan and top with sliced strawberries.

- Bake in preheated oven for 20-22 minutes.

- Serve and enjoy.

Per Serving: Net Carbs: 3.9g; Calories: 195; Total Fat: 17.7g; Saturated Fat: 6.4g Protein: 5.6g; Carbs: 5.9g; Fiber: 2g; Sugar: 0.9g; Fat 81% / Protein 11% / Carbs 8%

32.   Delicious Custard Tarts

<u>**Serves: 8**</u>

<u>**Preparation time: 10 minutes**</u>

<u>**Cooking time: 30 minutes**</u>

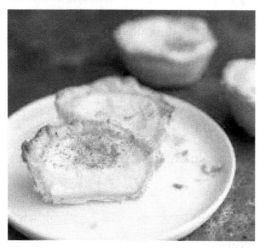

<u>**For crust:**</u>

- ¾ cup coconut flour

- 1 tbsp swerve

- 2 eggs

- ½ cup of coconut oil

- Pinch of salt

<u>**For custard:**</u>

- 3 eggs

- ½ tsp nutmeg

- 5 tbsp swerve

- 1 ½ tsp vanilla

- 1 ¼ cup unsweetened almond milk

Directions:

- For the crust: Preheat the oven to 400 F/ 200 C.

- In a bowl, beat eggs, coconut oil, sweetener, and salt.

- Add coconut flour and mix until dough is formed.

- Add dough in the tart pan and spread evenly.

- Prick dough with a knife.

- Bake in preheated oven for 10 minutes.

- For the custard: Heat almond milk and vanilla in a small pot until simmering.

- Whisk together eggs and sweetener in a bowl. Slowly add almond milk and whisk constantly.

- Strain custard well and pour into baked tart base.

- Bake in the oven at 300 F for 30 minutes.

- Sprinkle nutmeg on top and serve.

Per Serving: Net Carbs: 2.2g; Calories: 175; Total Fat: 17.2g; Saturated Fat: 12.9g Protein: 3.8g; Carbs: 2.9g; Fiber: 0.7g; Sugar: 0.4g; Fat 87% / Protein 8% / Carbs 5%

33. Easy Strawberry Pie

<u>**Serves: 8**</u>

<u>**Preparation time: 10 minutes**</u>

<u>**Cooking time: 10 minutes**</u>

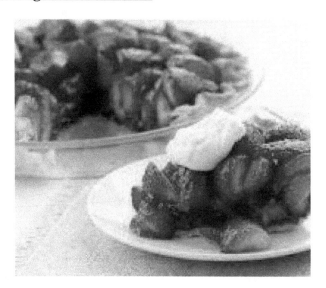

<u>For crust:</u>

- 2 tbsp butter, melted

- 1 cup pecans, chopped

- 1 tsp liquid stevia

<u>For filling</u>:

- ½ tsp vanilla

- 2/3 cup Swerve

- 1 cup strawberries, chopped

- 1 ½ cup heavy whipping cream

- 8 oz cream cheese, softened

Directions:

- Preheat the oven to 350 F/ 180 C.

- Add pecans in food processor and process until if finely crush.

- Add sweetener and butter in crushed pecans and process until well combined.

- Greased pie pan with butter.

- Add crust mixture into the greased pie pan and spread evenly. Using back of spoon smooth the pecan mixture.

- Bake in preheated oven for 10 minutes.

- Allow to cool completely.

- For the filling: In a large bowl, beat heavy whipping cream until stiff peaks form.

- In another bowl, add strawberries, vanilla, sweetener, and cream cheese and beat until smooth.

- Add heavy cream in strawberry mixture and beat until smooth.

- Pour strawberry cream mixture into crust and spread well.

- Place in refrigerator for 2 hours.

- Slice and serve.

Per Serving: Net Carbs: 3.1g; Calories: 314; Total Fat: 32.2g; Saturated Fat: 14.2g Protein: 4.3g; Carbs: 5g; Fiber: 1.9g; Sugar: 1.5g; Fat 92% / Protein 5% / Carbs 3%

Intermediate

34.   **Raspberry Tart**

<u>Serves: 4</u>

<u>Preparation time: 10 minutes</u>

<u>Cooking time: 23 minutes</u>

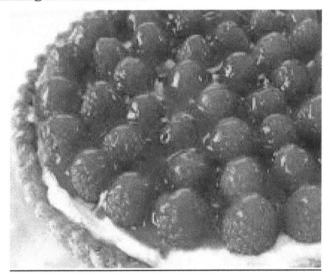

Ingredients:

- 5 egg whites

- 2 cups raspberries

- ½ cup butter, melted

- 1 tsp baking powder

- 1 tsp vanilla

- 1 lemon zest, grated

- 1 cup almond flour

- ½ cup xylitol

Directions:

- Preheat the oven to 375 F/ 190 C.

- Grease tart tin with cooking spray and set aside.

- In a large bowl, whisk egg whites until foamy.

- Add sweetener, baking powder, vanilla, lemon zest, and almond flour and mix until well combined.

- Add melted butter and stir well.

- Pour batter in prepared tart tin and top with raspberries.

- Bake in preheated oven for 20-23 minutes.

- Serve and enjoy.

Per Serving: Net Carbs: 4.2g; Calories: 213 Total Fat: 18.8g; Saturated Fat: 7.8g Protein: 5.8g; Carbs: 7.9g; Fiber: 3.7g; Sugar: 2.3g; Fat 81% / Protein 11% / Carbs 8%

35. Easy Lemon Pie

<u>Serves: 8</u>

<u>Preparation time: 10 minutes</u>

<u>Cooking time: 45 minutes</u>

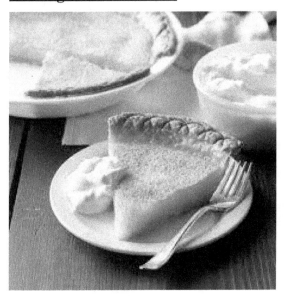

Ingredients:

- 3 eggs

- 3 lemon juice

- 1 lemon zest, grated

- 4 oz erythritol

- 5.5 oz almond flour

- 3.5 oz butter, melted

- Salt

Directions:

- Preheat the oven to 350 F/ 180 C.

- In a bowl, mix together butter, 1 oz sweetener, 3 oz almond flour, and salt.

- Transfer the dough in a pie dish and spread evenly and bake for 20 minutes.

- In a separate bowl, mix together eggs, lemon juice, lemon zest, remaining flour, sweetener, and salt.

- Pour egg mixture on prepared crust and bake for 25 minutes more.

- Allow to cool completely.

- Slice and serve.

Per Serving: Net Carbs: 3.0g; Calories: 229; Total Fat: 21.5g; Saturated Fat: 7.7g Protein: 6.5g; Carbs: 5.3g; Fiber: 2.3g; Sugar: 1.4g; Fat 84% / Protein 11% / Carbs 5%

36. Delicious Pumpkin Cream Pie

Serves: 10

Preparation time: 10 minutes

Cooking time: 60 minutes

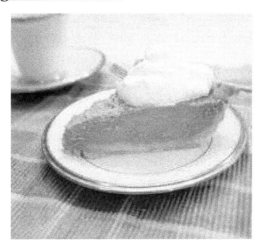

For crust:

- 1 tsp erythritol

- 8 tbsp butter

- 1 ¼ cup almond flour

- Pinch of salt

For filling:

- 2 eggs

- ½ tsp liquid stevia

- ½ cup erythritol

- 2 tbsp pumpkin pie spice

- ¼ cup sour cream

- ¾ cup heavy cream

- 15 oz can pumpkin puree

Directions:

- For the crust: Preheat the oven to 350 F/ 180 C.

- Add all crust ingredients into the food processor and process until dough is formed.

- Transfer the dough in a pie dish and spread evenly.

- Prick bottom on crust using fork or knife.

- Bake crust in preheated oven for 10 minutes.

- For the filling: Preheat the oven to 375 F/ 190 C.

- In a large bowl, whisk eggs with sour cream, heavy cream, and pumpkin puree.

- Add stevia, erythritol, and pumpkin pie spice and whisk well.

- Pour cream pumpkin mixture into the baked crust and spread evenly.

- Bake in preheated oven for 45-50 minutes.

- Allow to cool completely then place in the refrigerator for 2-3 hours.

- Serve and enjoy.

Per Serving: Net Carbs: 5.6g; Calories: 239; Total Fat: 21.8g; Saturated Fat: 9.5g Protein: 5.3g; Carbs: 8.3g; Fiber: 2.7g; Sugar: 2.1g; Fat 83% / Protein 8% / Carbs 9%

37. Strawberry Tart

Serves: 10

Preparation time: 15 minutes

Cooking time: 25 minutes

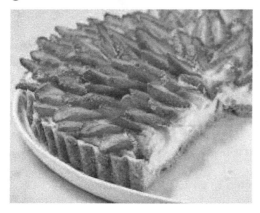

Ingredients:

- 1 egg

- 1/4 cup butter, melted

- 2 cups almond flour

- 1 tsp vanilla

- 1/4 cup Swerve

- For filling:

- 4 oz cream cheese

- 1 cup fresh strawberries, sliced

- 2 tbsp heavy cream

- 6 tbsp swerve

- 8 oz mascarpone cheese

- 1/2 tsp xanthan gum

- 1 tsp vanilla

Directions:

- Preheat the oven to 350 F/ 180 C.

- Spray the tart pan with cooking spray and set aside.

- For the crust: Add almond flour, vanilla, swerve, egg, and butter into the food processor and process until it forms into a dough.

- Transfer dough into the prepared tart pan.

- Spread dough evenly and lightly press down with your fingers.

- Prick crust dough with a knife and cover with parchment paper and dried beans.

- Bake in preheated oven for 20 minutes.

- Remove from oven and set aside to cool completely.

- For the filling: Add strawberries, heavy cream, swerve, vanilla, cream cheese, and mascarpone cheese into the food processor and process until smooth and creamy.

- Add xanthan gum and stir well.

- Pour filling mixture into baked crust and spread evenly.

- Place into the refrigerator for 1-2 hours.

- Slices and serve.

Per Serving: Net Carbs: 6.4g; Calories: 277 Total Fat: 24.3g; Saturated Fat: 8.9g Protein: 9g; Carbs: 9.3g; Fiber: 2.9g; Sugar: 1.7g; Fat 79% / Protein 12% / Carbs 9%

38. Butter Pie

Serves: 8

Preparation time: 15 minutes

Cooking time: 50 minutes

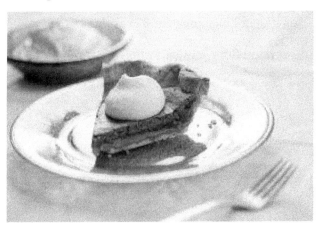

For crust:

- 1 egg

- 1/4 cup butter, melted

- 3 tbsp erythritol

- 1 1/4 cup almond flour

For filling:

- 1 egg

- 1 egg yolk

- 8 oz cream cheese, softened

- 1 cup butter, melted

- 1/2 cup erythritol

Directions:

- Preheat the oven to 375 F/ 190 C.

- Spray a 9-inch pie dish with cooking spray and set aside.

- For the crust: In a large bowl, mix together all crust ingredients until well combined.

- Transfer crust mixture into the prepared dish. Spread evenly and lightly press down with your fingers.

- Bake in preheated oven for 7 minutes.

- Remove from oven and set aside to cool completely.

- For the filling: In a mixing bowl, add all filling ingredients and mix using an electric mixer until well combined.

- Pour filling mixture into the crust and bake at 350 F/ 180 C for 35-40 minutes.

- Remove from oven and set aside to cool completely.

- Place in refrigerator for 1-2 hours.

- Slice and serve.

Per Serving: Net Carbs: 2.8g; Calories: 476 Total Fat: 49.1g; Saturated Fat: 25.6g Protein: 7.9g; Carbs: 4.7g; Fiber: 1.9g; Sugar: 0.8g; Fat 92% / Protein 6% / Carbs 2%

Expert

39. Crust-less Pumpkin Pie

<u>Serves: 4</u>

<u>Preparation time: 10 minutes</u>

<u>Cooking time: 30 minutes</u>

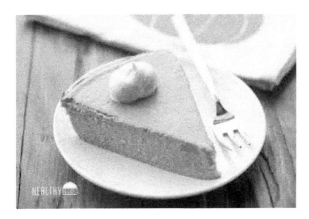

<u>Ingredients:</u>

- 3 eggs

- 1/2 cup cream

- 1/2 cup unsweetened almond milk

- 1/2 cup pumpkin puree

- 1/2 tsp cinnamon

- 1 tsp vanilla

- 1/4 cup Swerve

<u>Directions:</u>

- Preheat the oven to 350 F/ 180 C.

- Spray a square baking dish with cooking spray and set aside.

- In a large bowl, add all ingredients and whisk until smooth.

- Pour pie mixture into the prepared dish and bake in preheated oven for 30 minutes.

- Remove from oven and set aside to cool completely.

- Place into the refrigerator for 1-2 hours.

- Cut into the pieces and serve.

Per Serving: Net Carbs: 3.2g; Calories: 86; Total Fat: 5.5g; Saturated Fat: 2.1g Protein: 4.9g; Carbs: 4.4g; Fiber: 1.2g; Sugar: 2g; Fat 60% / Protein 25% / Carbs 15%

40.   Lemon Pie

Serves: 8

Preparation time: 10
minutes

Cooking time: 15
minutes

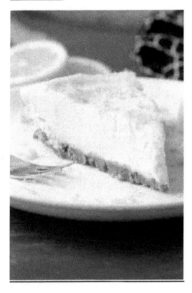

For crust:

- 1 cup pecans, chopped

- 1 tsp swerve

- 2 tbsp butter, melted

For filling:

- 1 tsp vanilla

- 1 1/2 cup heavy whipping cream

- 8 oz cream cheese, softened

- 2/3 cup Swerve

- 1/4 cup fresh lemon juice

- 1 tbsp lemon zest

Directions:

- Preheat the oven to 350 F/ 180 C.

- Add pecans into the food processor and process until pecans crush finely.

- Add swerve and butter into the crushed pecans and mix until well combined.

- Spray pie pan with cooking spray.

- Add crust mixture into the prepared pan.

- Spread evenly and lightly press down with your fingers.

- Bake in preheated oven for 10 minutes.

- Remove from oven and set aside to cool completely.

- For the filling: In a large bowl, beat whipping cream until stiff peaks forms.

- Add vanilla, swerve, and cream cheese and beat until smooth.

- Add lemon zest and lemon juice and beat until just combined.

- Pour filling mixture into the baked crust and spread evenly.

- Place in refrigerator for 1-2 hours. Slice and serve.

Per Serving: Net Carbs: 2.3g; Calories: 311 Total Fat: 32.2g; Saturated Fat: 14.3g Protein: 4.2g; Carbs: 3.9g; Fiber: 1.6g; Sugar: 0.9g; Fat 93% / Protein 5% / Carbs 2%

41. Coconut Pie

<u>**Serves: 8**</u>

<u>**Preparation time: 10 minutes**</u>

<u>**Cooking time: 20 minutes**</u>

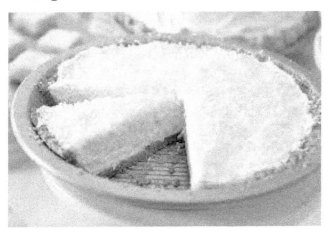

<u>**Ingredients:**</u>

- 2 oz shredded coconut

- 1/4 cup erythritol

- 1/4 cup coconut oil

- 5.5 oz coconut flakes

- 1 tsp xanthan gum

- 3/4 cup erythritol

- 2 cups heavy cream

<u>**Directions:**</u>

- Add coconut flakes, erythritol, and coconut oil into the food processor and process for 30-40 seconds.

- Transfer coconut flakes mixed into the pie pan and spread evenly.

- Lightly press down the mixture and bake at 350 F/ 180 C for 10 minutes.

- Heat heavy cream in a saucepan over low heat.

- Whisk in shredded coconut, powdered erythritol, and xanthan gum. Bring to boil.

- Remove from heat and set aside to cool for 10 minutes.

- Pour filling mixture onto the crust and place in the refrigerator for overnight.

- Slice and serve.

Per Serving: Net Carbs: 2.5g; Calories: 206; Total Fat: 21.4g; Saturated Fat: 15.9g Protein: 1.1g; Carbs: 3.8g; Fiber: 1.3g; Sugar: 1.7g; Fat 93% / Protein 3% / Carbs 4%

42. Apple Tart

Serves: 10

Preparation time: 10 minutes

Cooking time: 55 minutes

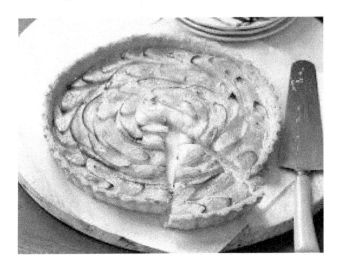

For crust:

- 2 cups almond flour

- 6 tbsp butter, melted

- 1/2 tsp cinnamon

- 1/3 cup erythritol

For filling:

- 1/4 cup erythritol

- 3 cups apples, peeled, cored, and sliced

- 1/2 tsp cinnamon

- 1/4 cup butter

- 1/2 tsp lemon juice

<u>Directions:</u>

- Preheat the oven to 375 F/ 190 C.

- For the crust: In a bowl, mix together butter, cinnamon, swerve, and almond flour until it lookscrumbly.

- Transfer crust mixture into the 10-inch spring-form pan and spread evenly using your fingers.

- Bake crust in preheated oven for 5 minutes.

- For the filling: In a bowl, mix together apple slices and lemon juice.

- Arrange apple slices evenly across the bottom of the baked crust in a circular shape.

- Press apple slices down lightly.

- In a small bowl, combine together butter, swerve, and cinnamon and microwave for 1 minute.

- Whisk until smooth and pour over apple slices.

- Bake tart for 30 minutes.

- Remove from oven and lightly press down apple slices with a fork.

- Turn heat to 350 F/ 180 C and bake for 20 minutes more.

- Remove from the oven and set aside to cool completely.

- Slice and serve.

Per Serving: Net Carbs: 3.7g; Calories: 236; Total Fat: 22.7g; Saturated Fat: 8.1g Protein: 5g; Carbs: 6.4g; Fiber: 2.7g; Sugar: 1.9g; Fat 86% / Protein 8% / Carbs 6%

43.   Mascarpone Tart

Serves: 10

Preparation time: 15 minutes

Cooking time: 20 minutes

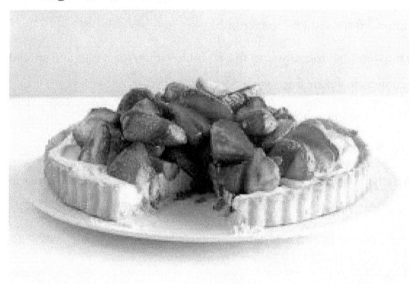

For crust:

- 1 egg

- 1/4 cup butter, melted

- 2 cups almond flour

- 1/2 tsp vanilla

- 1/4 cup Swerve

For filling:

- 6 oz mascarpone cheese

- 2 tbsp heavy cream

- 1/4 cup Swerve

- 3/4 cup lemon curd

Directions:

- Spray the tart pan with cooking spray and set aside.

- Preheat the oven to 350 F/ 180 C.

- Add almond flour, vanilla, swerve, egg, and butter into the food processor and process until it forms a dough.

- Add the dough into the prepared tart pan and spread out evenly.

- Prick the crust with a fork and cover with parchment paper and dried beans.

- Bake for 15 minutes.

- Remove from oven and set aside to cool completely.

- Add lemon curd, heavy cream, swerve, and mascarpone into the food processor and process until smooth and creamy.

- Pour filling mixture into the baked crust and spread evenly.

- Place in refrigerator for 2 hours.

- Slice and serve.

Per Serving: Net Carbs: 5.6g; Calories: 174 Total Fat: 17.4g; Saturated Fat: 8.4g Protein: 3.1g; Carbs: 6.2g; Fiber: 0.6g; Sugar: 5.1g; Fat 86% / Protein 5% / Carbs 9%

44. Flavorful Strawberry Cream Pie

Serves: 10

Preparation time: 10 minutes

Cooking time: 10 minutes

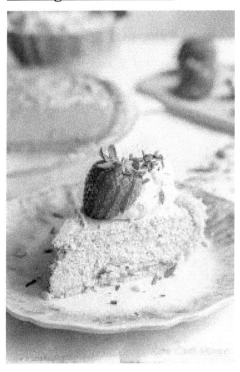

Ingredients:

- 1 cup almond flour

- ¼ cup butter, melted

- 8 oz cream cheese, softened

- ½ cup erythritol

- ½ cup fresh strawberries

- ¾ cup heavy whipping cream

Directions:

- In a bowl, mix together almond flour and melted butter.

- Spread almond flour mixture into the pie dish evenly.

- Add strawberries in a blender and blend until a smooth puree is formed.

- Add strawberry puree in a large bowl.

- Add remaining ingredients in a bowl and whisk until thick.

- Transfer Strawberry cream mixture onto the pie crust and spread evenly.

- Place in refrigerator for 2 hours.

- Slice and serve.

Per Serving: Net Carbs: 2.5g; Calories: 217; Total Fat: 21.5g; Saturated Fat: 10.4g Protein: 4.4g; Carbs: 3.8g; Fiber: 1.3g; Sugar: 0.8g; Fat 88% / Protein 8% / Carbs 4%

Candy

Beginner

45.   Strawberry Candy

<u>Serves: 12</u>

<u>Preparation time: 10 minutes</u>

<u>Cooking time: 10 minutes</u>

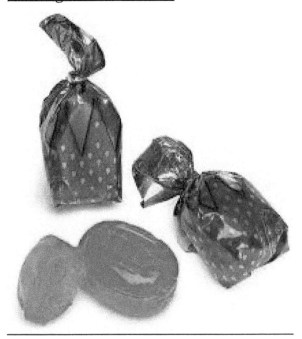

Ingredients:

- 3 fresh strawberries

- 1/2 cup butter, softened

- 8 oz cream cheese, softened

- 1/2 tsp vanilla

- 3/4 cup Swerve

<u>Directions:</u>

- Add all ingredients into the food processor and process until smooth.

- Pour mixture into the silicone candy mold and place in the refrigerator for 2 hours or until candy is hardened.

- Serve and enjoy.

Per Serving: Net Carbs: 0.8g; Calories: 136 Total Fat: 14.3g; Saturated Fat: 9g Protein: 1.5g; Carbs: 0.9g; Fiber: 0.1g; Sugar: 0.2g; Fat 94% / Protein 4% / Carbs 2%

46.   Blackberry Candy

<u>**Serves: 8**</u>

<u>**Preparation time: 5 minutes**</u>

<u>**Cooking time: 5 minutes**</u>

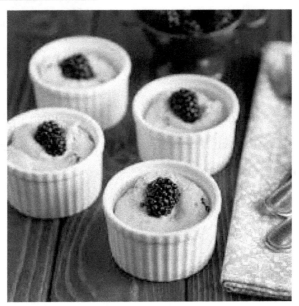

Ingredients:

- 1/2 cup fresh blackberries

- 1/4 cup cashew butter

- 1 tbsp fresh lemon juice

- 1/2 cup coconut oil

- ½ cup unsweetened coconut milk

Directions

- Heat cashew butter, coconut oil, and coconut milk in a pan over medium-low heat, until just warm.

- Transfer cashew butter mixture to the blender along with remaining ingredients and blend until smooth.

- Pour mixture into the silicone candy mold and refrigerate until set.

- Serve and enjoy.

Per Serving: Net Carbs: 2.9g; Calories: 203; Total Fat: 21.2g; Saturated Fat: 15.8g Protein: 1.9g; Carbs: 3.9g; Fiber: 1g; Sugar: 1g; Fat 92% / Protein 3% / Carbs 5%

47. Ginger Coconut Candy

Serves: 10

Preparation time: 5 minutes

Cooking time: 5 minutes

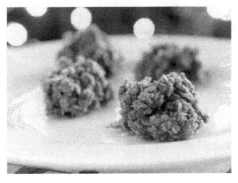

Ingredients:

- 1 tsp ground ginger

- 1/4 cup shredded coconut, unsweetened

- 3 oz coconut oil, softened

- 3 oz coconut butter, softened

- 1 tsp liquid stevia

Directions:

- Add coconut oil and coconut butter in a microwave-safe bowl and microwave for 30 seconds. Stir well.

- Add remaining ingredients and stir well to combine.

- Pour mixture into the silicone candy mold and refrigerate until hardened.

- Serve and enjoy.

Per Serving: Net Carbs: 0.8g; Calories: 130 Total Fat: 13.9g; Saturated Fat: 12.1g Protein: 0.6g; Carbs: 2.3g; Fiber: 1.5g; Sugar: 0.6g; Fat 96% / Protein 2% / Carbs 2%

48. Cocoa Butter Candy

<u>**Serves: 8**</u>

<u>**Preparation time: 5 minutes**</u>

<u>**Cooking time: 5 minutes**</u>

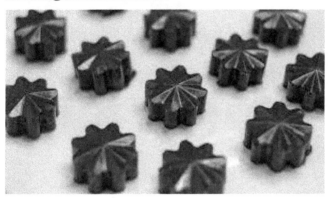

<u>**Ingredients:**</u>

- 1/4 cup cocoa butter

- 10 drops stevia

- 1/4 cup coconut oil

<u>**Directions:**</u>

- Melt together coconut oil and cocoa butter in a saucepan over low heat.

- Remove from heat and stir in stevia.

- Pour mixture into the silicone candy mold and refrigerate until hardened. Serve and enjoy.

Per Serving: Net Carbs: 0g; Calories: 119; Total Fat: 13.8g; Saturated Fat: 9.9g Protein: 0g; Carbs: 0g; Fiber: 0g; Sugar: 0g; Fat 100% / Protein 0% / Carbs 0%

49. Chocolate Candy

Serves: 10

Preparation time: 5 minutes

Cooking time: 10 minutes

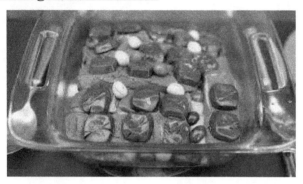

Ingredients:

- ½ cup of coconut oil

- ½ cup unsweetened cocoa powder

- ½ cup almond butter

- 1 tbsp stevia

- ½ tbsp sea salt

Directions:

- Melt coconut oil and almond butter in a saucepan and over medium heat.

- Add cocoa powder and sweetener and stir well.

- Remove pan from heat and let it cool for 5 minutes.

- Pour saucepan mixture in silicone candy mold and place in the refrigerator for 15 minutes or until set.

- Serve and enjoy.

Per Serving: Net Carbs: 1g; Calories: 109; Total Fat: 11.9g; Saturated Fat: 9.8g Protein: 1g; Carbs: 2.5g; Fiber: 1.5g; Sugar: 0.1g; Fat 98% / Protein 1% / Carbs 1%

Intermediate

50.   **Berry Cheese Candy**

Serves: 12

Preparation time: 5 minutes

Cooking time: 5 minutes

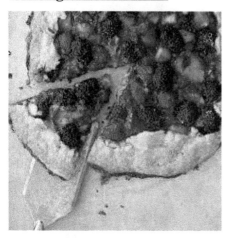

Ingredients:

- 1 cup fresh berries, wash

- 1/2 cup coconut oil

- 1 1/2 cup cream cheese, softened

- 1 tbsp vanilla

- 2 tbsp swerve

Directions:

- Add all ingredients to the blender and blend until smooth and combined.

- Spoon mixture into small candy molds and refrigerate until set.

- Serve and enjoy.

Per Serving: Net Carbs: 2.3g; Calories: 190; Total Fat: 19.2g; Saturated Fat: 14.2g Protein: 2.3g; Carbs: 2.7g; Fiber: 0.4g; Sugar: 1g; Fat 90% / Protein 5% / Carbs 5%

Recipe index

Easy Lemon Pie

Easy Strawberry Pie

Easy Peanut Butter Cookies

Flourless Chocó Cake

Fluffy Cookies

Flavorful Strawberry Cream Pie

Flavors Pumpkin Bars

Fudgy Chocolate Cake

Gingersnap Cookies

Ginger Coconut Candy

Gooey Chocolate Cake

Protein Bars

Peanut Butter Bars

Perfect Mint Ice Cream

Peanut Butter Ice Cream

Pumpkin Custard

Pecan Cookies

Lemon Cake

Lemon Cheesecake

Lemon Cheese Ice Cream

Lemon Pie

Mixed Berry Yogurt

Mascarpone Cheese Candy

Mascarpone Tart

Pumpkin Bars

Peanut Butter Pie

Pumpkin Candy

Peanut Butter

Pumpkin Cheesecake

Pumpkin Ice Cream

Raspberry Candy

Raspberry Tart Raspberry

Quick & Simple Strawberry

Strawberry Tart

Saffron Coconut Bars

Sesame Bars

Simple Chocolate Cookies

Sweet Blackberry Ice Cream

Strawberry Ice Cream

Strawberry Candy Strawberry

Yogurt Vanilla Butter Cake

Yogurt Raspberry Sorbet White

Chocolate Candy

Conclusion

A voiding dessert and labeling it as off-limits can lead to mental problems, according to science. Restrictive diets almost always have the opposite effects. Ironically, if you're trying not to think about desserts, you may even find yourself thinking about sweets all the time. You may end up daydreaming about a huge chocolate cake. For many people, avoiding the sweets they want may make their cravings even worse. This can lead to overeating and emotional stress.

When you enjoy a portion-controlled treat whenever you want, you will eat mindfully and ditch the guilt that causes stress and anxiety. Believe me, if you decide to enjoy dessert now and then, you'll be satisfied with fewer portions such as a small square of chocolate or a healthy protein smoothie. This approach will help you control your obsession with sweets. That sounds clichéd, but eating a balanced diet is the key to the ideal weight and overall health. Therefore, you should eat a healthy dessert not sugary desserts with "empty" calories. Numerous studies have found that eating dessert can help you eat less calories on a daily basis. What nutritionists eat for dessert? Their go-to dessert choices include dark chocolate, nuts, nut butter, fruits, and homemade energy bars.

CPSIA information can be obtained
at www.ICGtesting.com
Printed in the USA
BVHW070900150321
602550BV00010B/1067